IT'S NEVER TOO LATE SOMETIMES©

From health setbacks to success - A Family's odyssey

YVONNE STANBERRY

Co- Authors
Cleveland Stanberry
Antoinette Stanberry
Clive-Anthony Stanberry
Samantha Stanberry

Disclaimer

DEDICATION

To the incredibly devoted, educated, talented, and caring health workers that we were fortunate enough to meet starting in May 2003, plus supportive work colleagues, academics, families, and friends who enabled our family to navigate the sorrows and joys of life's journeys, reminding us that it's never too late sometimes, to move from trials to triumph.

ACKNOWLEDGMENTS

The support from many individuals cannot be overstated. They helped in numerous ways to transform our aspirations into this book.

The moral support of our family's educational achievements from Beverley Igbinosun and Onilla (Maureen) Bailey provided the catalyst to get the writing underway. Our motivation was heightened after they hosted a celebratory, educational achievement party in our honor.

Sophia Lewis of the "Long Story Short Podcast" immediately understood our vision of the book the moment we shared it with her. She wasted no time in introducing us to Dr. Ava Eagle Brown.

Dr. Ava Eagle Brown's Book2Biz Publishing services provided invaluable editing, layout, and formatting recommendations and services that resulted in this polished work.

We owe a debt of gratitude to each of the people mentioned in the book; they played stellar roles that led us to this stage of our twisting journey.

We extend our deepest gratitude to the remarkable Dr. Joan Y. Lyn, Dr. Molapo Selepe, and Rebecca Leach, who generously provided endorsements for this book. Your thoughtful and inspiring words have added immense value, and your support of our family has been a guiding light throughout our journeys. Thank you for sharing your expertise in your respective disciplines and lending your voice to this endeavor.

Praise for It's Never Too Late Sometimes©

It's Never Too Late Sometimes© - is a powerful testament to the resilience of the human spirit and the strength of family bonds in the face of unimaginable challenges. As a physician, I am acutely aware of the immense anxiety that accompanies a diagnosis of Aplastic Anemia, especially when a child's platelet count falls below 10—an experience that can be deeply distressing for informed, concerned parents. This gripping memoir follows the Stanberry family's journey from the brink of a life-threatening crisis to the incredible educational accomplishments that stemmed from their unwavering determination and unity. Their story is both heart-wrenching and inspiring, demonstrating that even in the darkest moments, hope, love, and perseverance can lead to extraordinary outcomes. A truly moving and inspiring read."

Dr. Joan Y. Lyn, DO., MPH. Board-certified family practice physician in North Miami Beach, Florida.

"The Stanberry family's journey is an inspiring testament to the power of a resolute sense of resilience and perseverance. When circumstances so easily dictated that they wallow in the depths of despair and the comfort of despondency they held onto hope and extraordinary courage. It beggars belief how they faced their ordeal with such profound poise and prowess. It was as if there was an unseen presence and reassurance, that infused their lives with wisdom and clarity of thought to make the right decisions that shaped them into champions.

Moving from the frightening reality of an Aplastic Anemia diagnosis to achieving seven University of London degrees as a family is a truly extraordinary feat. As someone familiar with the University of London's high academic rigor and exceptional standards, I am in awe of their collective and individual accomplishments. This memoir beautifully showcases how, even in the darkest times, a shared vision and sound familial support can lead to psychological and spiritual resilience.

The unparalleled academic success of the Stanberry family speaks to the dire need in our society right now, that of a role of a stable and intact family in one's overall success in life. A compelling and riveting story of the transformative power of trusting in your own journey. In this case we learn how the Stanberrys knew that it's never too late for anyone to follow their hopes and dreams even in the face of seemingly impossible odds stacked against them."

Dr. Molapo Selepe, MD, Family Physician in Perth, Australia.

Author of "A New Afrikan Trilogy", "The Extra Mile".

"The Stanberry family's journey from facing the life-altering diagnosis of Aplastic Anemia to achieving seven University of London degrees is a truly extraordinary story of perseverance, unity, and triumph. Having worked alongside Cleveland for nearly two decades and knowing the family for that period, I have witnessed firsthand the incredible dedication and resilience they bring to every endeavor. This memoir is a powerful reminder that even the most daunting obstacles can be transformed into remarkable accomplishments with determination and strong family support. An inspiring read for anyone seeking motivation and hope."

Rebecca Leach, CLC, Technology Executive and Leadership Coach.

Former Country Leader of AppDynamics, and General Manager of Cisco Software Sales.

PREFACE

Our family decided to write this book because one of us was affected by a rare disease that initially appeared to be cancer. Based on patient observation, platelet count, red and white blood counts, other results from complete blood count tests, and medical clinicians' assessments, it was first thought to be leukemia.

However, after a successful bone marrow aspirate biopsy and subsequent investigation, the medical team concluded and confirmed the diagnosis to be **Aplastic Anemia**. That diagnosis would soon evolve to a more severe form of the disease, sometimes referred to as **Acute Aplastic Anemia** or **Severe Acute Aplastic Anemia**. Throughout this book, we mostly refer to the disease simply as Aplastic Anemia.

We found that when sharing about Aplastic Anemia with people we encountered in life—including some trained healthcare professionals—many struggled to understand what we were talking about. Responses often included: "Oh, my brother is anemic, so he takes iron supplements," "It's best to eat red meat because that boosts your red blood cell count," or "Most people get over anemia with a good diet."

Not once, in 20 years, has anyone asked us what **'Aplastic'** means. That word was usually ignored. In our simple understanding, we took Aplastic to mean "not plastic," in the same way we interpret **'Atypical'** as meaning "not typical" or "not the norm."

When we first heard the term Aplastic Anemia from the attending physicians, we associated it with "not-typical anemia," only to later realise that we were in the same clinic as patients being treated for diseases such as leukemia and myelodysplasia. We wondered why were we there alongside patients with such dreaded, life-altering diseases. It turns out that Aplastic Anemia is also a dreaded, life-altering disease. We eventually learned that Aplastic Anemia is more closely related to leukemia than to the common understanding of anemia, which involves low red blood cell counts.

We fully understand that most people wouldn't have access to the information we've gained about Aplastic Anemia. This lack of understanding contributes to the difficulty people have in grasping its severity and the challenges involved in treating it successfully. Nonetheless, it was painful and frustrating to deal with the responses we received.

When trying to explain the seriousness of the disease with our limited knowledge, we would often state that Aplastic Anemia isn't caused by low red blood cells or iron deficiency, but that it's dangerous because of extremely low platelet counts. That's where we would often lose people. At the time, we had only just learned about platelets and their critical functions in the body through our experience with the disease. We understood that most people hadn't had the same education we received while sitting beside our loved one's hospital bed.

The distinctions between **Leukemia**, **Aplastic Anemia**, and **Anemia** are outlined in the table below. It is clear that leukemia and Aplastic Anemia are generally much more severe diseases.

Parts of the Blood	Leukemia	Aplastic Anemia	Anemia
White blood cells	Bone marrow makes abnormal cells that don't fight infections	Bone marrow makes abnormal cells that don't fight infections	Normal levels
Platelets	Bone marrow makes less platelets than are needed - can lead to bleeding easily	Bone marrow makes less platelets than are needed - can lead to bleeding easily	Normal levels
Red blood cells	Bone marrow cannot make enough red blood cells	Bone marrow cannot make enough red blood cells	Red blood cell count is low
	Treatment include bone marrow transplants, immunotherapy (medications to lower immune system function), chemotherapy, radiation)	Treatment includes bone marrow transplants or immunotherapy (medications to lower immune system function)	Treatment includes added Supplements such as: - Iron - Folic acid Vitamin B12

Sources:

- https://www.hopkinsmedicine.org/health/conditions-and-diseases/aplastic-anemia

- https://www.nhlbi.nih.gov/health/anemia/aplastic-anemia

- https://www.mayoclinic.org/diseases-conditions/leukemia/symptoms-causes/syc-20374373

- https://www.yalemedicine.org/conditions/anemia

We hope that this book will explain our journey with Aplastic Anemia in plain terms, its severity, the treatment regime that we accepted and how we are still hopeful for continued longer-term satisfactory health outcomes after more than twenty years of diagnosis. Explaining the severity or full meaning of Aplastic Anemia is outside of the capabilities of the authors. Rather, we will focus on our experiences of the disease, and how a family member with the disease moved from childhood to adulthood.

We will paint the picture of the family's obsession with high educational achievement and end the book with what they all accomplished despite what they thought was initially a gloomy outlook. We trust that the book appeals to those who might be looking for hope for a loved one who is being treated for Aplastic Anemia or any similarly devastating diagnosis.

Appeal to:

- Those who want to be inspired to know that we can move from despair through tragedy to triumph

- People who want to believe that we can move from dungeons to deliverance

- Individuals who can be motivated to transition from the focus on impossibilities to bask in the promise of hope

- Families who need to gaze their thoughts away from the darkest depths of despair and embrace the belief of a brighter future

- Non-fiction readers who widely share memoirs of hope with others to lift the spirit of humankind

- Families who are passionate about positive health and education outcomes

The book is purposely short so that it can be read within five hours. We believe that it could provide the fuel for inspiration if one were to read it on a flight from New York to Los Angeles, from Toronto to Vancouver, from New York to London, from Jamaica to Chicago. On a train ride across the country, cuddling up on a seat with a fruit juice in hand, or enjoying warm waves coming off the beachfront.

The book has five authors, all members of the same family - mother, father, twin sisters and their brother. Through their unique lenses, they each offer their experiences through their schooling, against the backdrop of dealing with Aplastic Anemia. We trust that each sentence was written in a clear and simple manner that allows for quick inspiration that can drive the reader to taking the steps to reach their aspirational goals.

For further comprehensive information about Aplastic Anemia, please visit:

A. SickKids Hospital,
   https://www.sickkids.ca/en/staff/d/yigal-dror/

   a. SickKids QR Code

B. Aplastic Anemia & Myelodysplasia Association of Canada (AAMAC), https://aamac.ca/

    a. AAMAC QR Code

C. National Institute of Health (NIH), USA https://www.niddk.nih.gov/health-information/blood-diseases/aplastic-anemia-myelodysplastic-syndromes

    a. NIH QR Code

D. National Health Service (NHS), Great Ormond Street Hospital for Children, UK, https://www.gosh.nhs.uk/conditions-and-treatments/conditions-we-treat/aplastic-anaemia/

    a. NHS QR Code

Contents

1

The Voice – The Clock Is Ticking

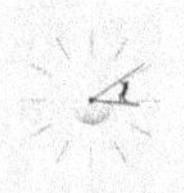

It was a voice unlike any other!

With a calm dogmatic demeanor the voice directed the message to me as both an order and as information sharing; information shared with me that I somehow knew, deep within my gut, that I had to act on. The words in the message I heard were nerve-wracking and could've easily sent spills shivering down my spine. Yet still, I was calm, but with a deep sense that at this very moment, I had to take charge of whatever was directed at my family.

For my husband and I, it was our norm to pray, plan, and effectively execute decisions once they were made. If we lived by any decision-making methodology mantras, this would have been one of them. We had already decided the next steps in the management of what we thought were harmless-looking red spots on Samantha's skin.

So, when I heard the words, "Samantha is sick, and the clock is ticking," it jerked me from the usually well-laid plans that we had in place to that moment's jarring reality. On this spring day, at about 7:00 AM, Thursday, May 15, 2003, we had already secured an appointment and planned to take Samantha to her Pediatrician the upcoming Saturday, May 17, 2003. Dr. Duic, the pediatrician, was well respected in the medical community. We were comfortably awaiting to visit his clinic, and like many, we had complete confidence in him due to his well-known expertise. This carefully crafted plan was about to go awry.

Only moments after I heard the chilling words, two of my three children came running into my bedroom. I asked my son, "Where's Samantha?" and he said, "She's sleeping." I told him to go and wake her. Samantha is the firstborn of twin girls. He left to wake her, and soon, they both scurried back into the room.

Much earlier, about 5:30 AM, my husband had left for the airport to catch a flight to Ottawa for a business trip for the day, expecting to return home that evening. This was a regular part of his routine, so nothing was unusual in our day so far. What was unusual was the jarring reverberation in my head, "Samantha is sick, and the clock is ticking." With him out of reach, I knew it was up to me to decide what next steps to take. I needed to respond and effectively deal with what lay ahead. There was no doubt in my head that the words that I knew I heard and the gut feeling that I had, were for me and the speaker of those words, a private communication that needed courses of action in public spaces and assistance that didn't include my husband.

Sometimes, I ponder and purposefully weigh options prior to decision-making. This morning was not to be one of those times. I telephoned our family doctor, Dr. Kebede, whose practice at the time didn't have too many patients, so it was usually easy to get an appointment. If memory serves me well, I was told by the receptionist to come in at 10:30 am. Having secured the appointment, using my landline telephone, I called my mother's landline phone. She lived about ten minutes away by car, so I asked her to come over and babysit my son and another daughter. I didn't tell her about the voice that gave me the message. I thought that that would be too irrational to share. Furthermore, the conversation with the 'voice' was, for me, a private conversation.

Mom arrived within thirty minutes, and this gave me ample time to get us ready to make the thirty-minute drive to the family doctor. While getting ready for the journey, I convinced myself that this was a form of due diligence because we had already secured an appointment two days away with one of the most notable pediatricians in the city. So, there was nothing to lose by hopping over to visit the family doctor. This seemed like the most rational thing any mother would do.

Knowing that I heard that Samantha was sick and the clock was ticking interestingly kept me calm and composed. But what does the clock ticking really mean to me? At that moment, for me, it meant that my reason for booking the appointment to see the pediatrician was just a small symptom of a much larger problem. And, furthermore, I might not have enough time left before the upcoming appointment on Saturday before the clock stops ticking. But whose clock would that be? Samantha's clock?

While driving our minivan to the family doctor's office, I calmly assured myself that although the clock might be ticking, I was doing something about it. I was not going to idly sit around and do nothing when I was audibly warned by an unknown voice that the clock "is ticking." "I am going to beat that clock," I thought.

The drive to the family doctor was within the expected thirty minutes. I went through the usual routine of submitting

Samantha's health card and other administrative formalities, including address, phone number, and other information. I was then asked to take a seat along with the others in the waiting room. The waiting room had about ten people seated and the office hosts about three doctors, so I assumed that they were not all there to see my family doctor. About fifteen minutes after sitting, I was called to another private room, where Samantha and I sat for another ten minutes.

Dr. Kebede walked in and said, in his usual pleasant Ethiopian accent, "Good morning, how are you? And how is the family?" The question was not surprising because, at that time, my family had been patients of Dr. Kebede for three to four years, so he knew of us. "The family is doing well, but I brought in Samantha because I saw some small spots and some bruises on her body," I replied.

Now, is that the true reason that I brought her in, I thought. That was somewhat true, but I knew I brought her in because I heard the 'voice,' and the words of that 'voice' were crystal clear. But could I ever be considered credible if I gave him that reason? In the most inner quiet sanctum of my purest thoughts, I believe the correct answer is 'no.' That is not a story to share with my family doctor, I concluded. I didn't even share it with my mother earlier in the day, so why share it with him, I thought.

"Where on her body are the spots and bruises?" Dr. Kebede asked. "Some small red spots are on her arms and on her back, and there is one large bruise on her belly," I responded. There were perhaps ten pen-tip-sized bruises on each of her arms and about fifty of the same size scattered across her back. They were slightly red and about 1 millimeter in diameter. The large bruise on her belly was somewhat oval, shaped like an island basking in sunshine in the Caribbean Sea, measuring about one centimeter wide by two centimeters long at their biggest points.

As I spoke, he took notes. "And when was the first time that you saw these bruises?" he asked. "About a week ago," I said. He put away his notes, washed his hands, and then asked me to lay Samantha on her back on the examination table. Next, he looked at the tiny bruises on her arms and then asked me to roll her face down. He glided his hands over the multiple pencil-tip-sized spots on her back in silence. My next job was to roll her face up so that he could examine the bruise on her abdomen. Once that was done, he looked at the bruise, gently touched it, and glided his hands over it, seemingly checking for any reaction from Samantha. She didn't flinch or move.

My next role was to put Samantha's clothes back together and take her from the table. She sat in my lap. He washed his hands, sat on the chair facing us, and said, "I would like to do some blood work and see the results. However, if I order the tests, it will take days for me to get the results. So, I will write a letter for you to take to the Mississauga Trillium Hospital Emergency Department. They can do the tests and will get back the results within hours rather than days". He left the room for less than ten minutes and returned with the letter to take to Mississauga's Trillium Hospital at 100 Queensway W – at the corner of Hurontario Street and The Queensway W in Mississauga.

About a week before I heard the voice, my husband and I saw the spots and the bruises and quizzed the children about Samantha falling, hitting herself on the dresser, or whether they were still jumping from the chest of drawers. To this day, they said none of these things happened. To be fully transparent, if I were not the caregiver, I would have assumed that whoever was caring for her used a blunt object to stab her in the abdomen. Later, I would come to understand from other doctors and parents that some parents were charged and jailed for similar bruises on their young children because of similar bruises observed when they were brought in to see their doctors. I came to realize that I was fortunate to have a family doctor who could spot what was truly going on.

*** Hospital One ***

Fortunately, the drive to the hospital was only about fifteen minutes. I knew the location of this hospital well because it was where my twin girls were born two years earlier. But, for whatever reason, once I got there, I could not find the visitors' parking lot. After a few minutes of trying to find it, I saw that the arm of a parking area was opened and pointing vertically. It is unusual for the arm to move vertically before the vehicle reaches it, but at that moment, I was just relieved that I could park and get to the emergency area. So, I drove in and parked in one of the spots.

We came out of the minivan, and I walked to a locked door that opened the minute we approached. A pleasant man pushed it wider for us to enter. The place looked different from the usual entrance to the emergency section of hospitals that I momentarily wondered how this could be happening, especially since I was familiar with this building. I brushed the thought aside and asked the man for directions to the emergency registration area. For some odd reason, I also showed him the letter. He read it and pointed to an area not far from the door - it was the emergency registration area.

I followed his instructions, and we arrived at the emergency registration desk. I went to the registration desk, informed the nurse of my letter from Dr. Kebede, handed her the letter, and provided the health card and the usual information. She put a registration card around Samantha's wrist, which reminded me of passes that one would get to enter a concert. She read the letter and asked me to wait in one of the seats. She got up from the desk and walked away out of my sight. I didn't know exactly what was written in the letter, but I suspected that it gave instructions to conduct blood tests, as Dr. Kebede told me earlier that morning.

As expected, we waited for a moment - perhaps five or ten minutes - before the nurse returned and called me to the desk. She then directed us through a door to a room down a hallway. Just a few moments after sitting in this room, another nurse entered with what looked like small trays in her hands and announced that she would be taking blood for a CBC. The only CBC that I knew was the Canadian Broadcasting Corporation, but I didn't think that's what she meant by that acronym. That same day, I would come to learn that within the medical context, CBC is the acronym for Complete Blood Count. I would continue to hear that term for the next seventeen years. Sometimes, I, too, would fluently use the acronym five times per week in conversations with hospital staff. Wow, it's never too late sometimes© to learn something new.

Like most nurses who feel called to the profession, she tried to make Samantha comfortable and told her to look away at an object in the room. She tied the elastic band around her arm and asked me to hold her steadily in my lap. As she looked for the vein in Samantha's hand (right hand, I think) and approached the vein with the needle, Samantha turned around, looked at the needle, and pulled her hand away with excessive force. I could not hold her still. She cried profusely. I suppose she had no intention of that thing piercing her flesh.

The nurse left and returned with straps that were used to restrain her. There might have been three or four across her body across the bed on which she was laid. She anxiously stared at the needle as the red liquid moved from her arm to the first vial. The nurse expertly removed one vial and inserted another and another. Three vials of blood were taken from one small child; these were the thoughts going through my mind. This was difficult for me to watch, but somehow, I knew it had to be done because I believed that "Samantha is sick, and the clock is ticking." Once completed, the nurse asked us to return to the waiting area until we were called.

It must have been 1:00 PM or 1:30 PM by now. Since Dr. Kebede told me that the hospital would get the blood test results back within hours, I knew that we wouldn't get home in under an hour. So, I used this opportunity to call home and check in on how things were going and to update Mom on my movements from Dr. Kebede's office to the hospital. As soon as she answered my call, I gave her an update. She told me that my husband had called earlier, and she informed him that I had taken Samantha to see the family doctor because of the red spots and bruises. I told her to tell him that I was at the hospital when he called back. I knew that he would keep calling to find out what was happening because that's one of his faults – he likes to follow up with things until the very end. He's an intense person who does not let anything go to rest until he's satisfied that it's completed. He has a strange likeness to the Greek word Telos, which he says means irreversible completed. He couldn't call me directly because back in 2003, cell phones were not in widespread use, at least not by most of the people that I knew. So, I expected he would use the cell phone that he had for work to keep checking in to get updates.

Forty-five minutes or more must have passed since the blood was transferred from the vein to the vials, so we went to get lunch in the food court. It wasn't much of a food court. There was a coffee shop and another food shop that sold sandwiches. Samantha was not a picky eater, so it was easy to get her something to eat. We ate, and afterward, Samantha did what she loved to do - jump. We were in a quiet area of the open food court, so I allowed her to enjoy jumping for a few minutes. Now, I thought it was time to return to the waiting area.

We sat and waited for another few hours, I think. When we were called to see the doctor, it must have been about 5:00 PM. We were escorted past the vein-to-vial room, through a door, and into the doctor's office. Dr Taylor was pleasant and easy to talk to, as was evident in her first words to me. "Good afternoon, Mother. I am Dr Taylor", she greeted me. "Good afternoon," I replied. "How did you know that you should bring her in?" she asked.

This question poured a bucket of confusion over me because, up to this point, I didn't know the seriousness of the situation that my daughter was in. Even though confusion was my silent partner at the time, I knew that I couldn't start babbling about hearing a voice. That didn't seem sane in this setting. Now, if I randomly surveyed one hundred people and asked if they were in my position, how many would state that they brought her in because they heard a voice saying, "Samantha is sick, and the clock is ticking"? The reasonable answer, I believe, is zero. And I believe that would be statistically valid!

"How did I know that I should bring her in?" I repeated. "I didn't know that I should bring her in," I said. "I saw spots and a bruise on her, and we made an appointment to see her pediatrician this Saturday, but I felt I should take her to our family doctor this morning. And he gave me a letter to come here and do blood tests to figure out what caused the spots", I rambled, trying not to divulge the true reason. "You did very well to take her to see him," she assured me. "So, who do you live with at home?" she asked. "My husband and our other two children," I replied.

My replies most likely came out as questions because I never recall being questioned like this by a healthcare provider. Despite the thoughts swirling in my mind regarding why these questions were being directed my way, I soon realized that Dr. Taylor's warm demeanor reflected her concern for the welfare of the entire family, as she intended for me to embark on yet another journey, away from home.

She said that she had another letter for me. Unbeknownst to me, she said that she had called the SickKids Hospital and asked if she should start treatment. SickKids Hospital said no, she shouldn't. They told her that she should let the child come to them immediately.

This letter now, in my possession, is to be taken to the SickKids Hospital in Toronto. "Don't stop; go straight there," she said. By this time, she got up from her desk and said that I should leave now. She opened her door, showed us out, and led us along the hallway.

As we passed by the vein-to-vial room, Dr. Taylor asked, "Who is now with your other children? "My mother," I answered. "And would your husband be able to meet you here?" she asked. "I don't think so; he flew to Ottawa this morning on business and is not expected to arrive home before the 6:00 PM flight", I informed her. We walked towards the door at the end of the hallway that leads to the emergency waiting area. She opened the door, and I blurted out with the same excitement that I would see people playing bingo on TV, "There he is!"

My husband, Cleveland, was walking towards the same door that we were exiting. Dr. Taylor brought him up to speed on what she thought was happening and told him, "We think it's cancer that your daughter has, but we don't have the expertise and experience to treat her. The SickKids Hospital has staff with the know-how and techniques to manage her. You should go there now, and don't stop".

We thanked Dr. Taylor and made our way to the minivan. I directed Cleveland to where I parked, and his surprising question was, "How did you get in here?" "The arm of the gate was opened, and I drove in," I said. "This is staff parking; you should need a staff pass to get into this space. See, there's the machine for the fob", Cleveland said as he pointed. "Did you pay for parking?" he asked. "No", I replied. "This is all so strange, I don't know why the arm was up so you could drive in without a fob. Perhaps a car was ahead of you, and you drove in before it went horizontal", he said.

What he didn't know was that not only did the parking arm stay vertical, allowing us to drive in, but earlier that day, I heard "the voice." He would later learn all about that. I was now more convinced, far more than ever, that this day was no normal day. How on earth did the arms go up to get me into the staff parking that led me to a door adjacent to the emergency registration desk?

We now needed to travel to another registration desk in another hospital. This time, the distance was much farther away. The distance to the SickKids Hospital is about twenty-five kilometers (15.5 miles) away. With rush hour traffic at approximately 5:00 PM this would take us more than an hour. We were determined to get there, so Cleveland first buckled our daughter into the car seat, secured his backpack that contained his work laptop into the back of the minivan, checked if we had enough gas in the van, and started the vehicle to go on yet another phase of this very unusual day. I was very interested to know how he ended up at the hospital. So, while on our way, he got me up to speed on how he ended up at the hospital and walking towards the door from which we were exiting.

Now that I understood why he was on the other side of that door, I told him about how the day started with the 'voice' and the chain of events that followed. I had a sense of great relief to be able to talk with someone about the 'voice' because up to this point, I didn't dare mention it to anyone.

But for Cleveland, how was his day?

***** Hospital Two *****

My day started like any other business day. At that stage of my life, my job required me to travel extensively, so the family would be familiar with me leaving the house in a cab at 5:30 to the airport on a Monday morning and returning on Thursday or Friday evening. Sometimes, like it was on May 15, 2003, I would be gone for only a day, landing back in Toronto by 6:00 PM. I purposefully schedule my day trips this way because it allows me to take the thirty-minute Airport Limousine ride home, shower, and have dinner with the family.

When I left Toronto's Pearson Airport on Thursday morning, I caught my usual Air Canada 7:30 AM flight, which got me into Ottawa at 8:30 AM. On my laptop, I reviewed my presentation file while I sat in the back of the Ottawa taxi. The Ottawa traffic was a bit heavier than normal this morning, so when I arrived at the hotel's conference center, where I was presenting a training course, I had no time to call home to let my wife know that I had arrived safely. I thought to myself that I'd just call her at lunchtime.

Presenting to large groups of people is something that I love to do, and this day was no different. The information technology networking content that I was presenting was one that I had delivered to many audiences across Canada, from Vancouver to Montreal, several times over, so the material was one that I tweaked to my likeness and could vary the pace based on the attendees' response. The first half of the session up to lunch went smoothly, and we broke for lunch a few minutes after noon.

Before eating the lunch, catered by the hotel, placed on tables at the back of the conference room, I called home to update Yvonne that all was going well. 'Chirp,' 'chirp,' 'chirp,' the phone rang back in my ears. And then, I heard "Hello". 'This voice is not Yvonne's voice,' was my split-second thought. I knew the voice, but that wasn't a problem. I was thinking, why isn't Yvonne answering the phone? Yvonne's mom, Pauline, answered the call, and I said, "Good afternoon, you're visiting the grandkids." "Not really", she said, "Yvonne called me this morning because she had to take Samantha to the doctor, and he sent her to Trillium Hospital Emergency for blood tests." In that split second, for no rational reason, I said to myself, 'Samantha has Cancer!'. It was not logical; there was no basis for this thinking. However, I now believe that the thought of Cancer was to prepare me for what Dr. Taylor would later say to me that evening.

Having been jerked by this thought, I asked Pauline about the other two children, and she assured me that they were doing well, eating and playing. I ended the call, but I didn't even ask if our son went to school that morning. Being two years old, our daughters were not yet enrolled in school, but he was. I was now focused on getting out of Ottawa. But I had a duty to these people who had set aside their day to attend my session. I had to develop a plan that would work well for them and me. Sometimes, I thought, "One must air their sad stories to others".

So, after I quickly ate something, I asked everyone in the room if they were okay if we started before the lunch hour was up. I told them that I had just heard that my wife was at the hospital with one of our daughters, sent there by the family doctor to have blood work done. Also, I asked if we could cut the usual afternoon fifteen-minute break so that I could leave early. Every single person in the room agreed, and within moments, we resumed the session.

I ended the session at about 2:30 PM, hoping that if all went well, I could get on a 3:00 PM flight. That was not to be because the afternoon Ottawa traffic was so heavy that I arrived at the airport at 3:30 PM. I missed the 3:30 flight and got a seat on the 4:00 PM flight. This was the first time ever, that I missed a flight that I intended to get on. This route was a regular one for me, so there were several occasions when I timed my meetings to get out on an earlier flight, so I thought I knew well how to game the schedule. Not this time, however.

After landing at Toronto Pearson Airport an hour later, I ran into the Airport Limousine black car at the front of the queue and instructed the driver to head to the Mississauga Trillium Hospital on the Queensway. The traffic on Highway 401 was cooperating much more than the Ottawa traffic. Within almost twenty minutes, I arrived at the hospital's emergency entrance, at which I instructed the driver to stop. I swiftly paid by credit card and bolted from the car. I went to the registration desk and told the nurse sitting there that I was looking for my wife and daughter and gave their names. She was aware of who they were and pointed me toward a door. I thanked her and immediately started walking in that direction. I might have been twenty feet away when the door swung open in front of me, and I saw Yvonne's finger pointing at me and heard her shouting, "There he is!". This was strange, I thought to myself. Obviously, they were talking about me, but how could they be expecting to see me here?

Yvonne's recount of her day was vivid, and it sounded more like a dream, a novel, or a movie rather than actual events that she had witnessed. But by now, we were driving to SickKids hospital, so her day was real because I - my ears and my own voice - was now a part of her reality, driving from Mississauga to Toronto's SickKids hospital.

To this day, I remain convinced that on the morning of May 15, 2003, I needed to be away from Yvonne's physical space and unreachable by phone. This gave her the courage, I believe, to make good independent decisions, the right decisions that resulted in taking the best actions that started the ball rolling on finding the solutions beneficial to Samantha's health outcome. She didn't need me to distract her from doing what she did best.

2

The Admission

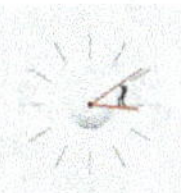

The journey from Mississauga's Trillium Hospital, as it was called then, was a twenty-five-kilometer journey, as seen in the map below.

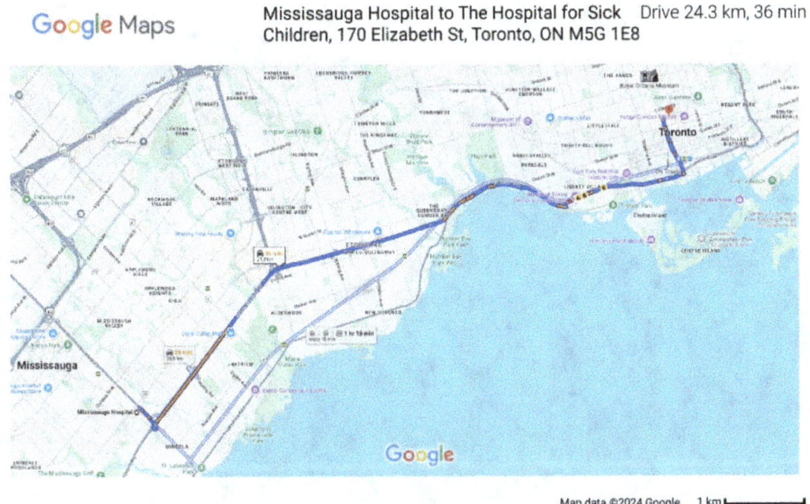

Source: https://www.google.com/maps

This traffic was not the heaviest that I've seen it, so we arrived in downtown Toronto in about an hour. Upon arriving for the first time ever at the SickKids Hospital address at 555 University Avenue, Toronto, and while we were still in the minivan, I quickly realized that this was not the emergency entrance. Neither was there parking at this location. This was clearly constructed as a "kiss and ride" drop-off location. Our mental state was certainly not in a "kiss and ride" mode, so I read as many of the signs and instructions posted on the outside of the building, and these pointed us towards Elizabeth Street, number 170, to be exact. The drive from 555 University Avenue to the emergency department meant making only right turns - one on Gerrard Street West and a right on the perpendicular-running Elizabeth Street. So, the one-block-away drive took us under five minutes. We located and pulled into the emergency department below the large Emergency sign. The map below displays the route from 555 University Avenue to 170 Elizabeth Street.

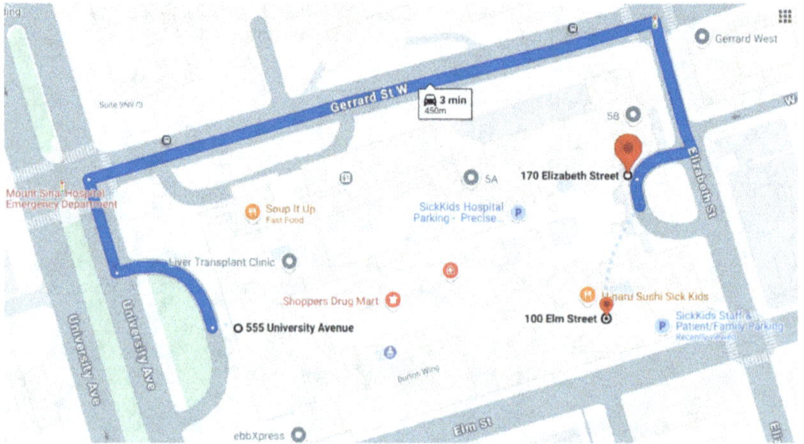

Source: https://www.google.com/maps

During this short drive, I pondered thoughts that seemed to have taken up an hour of my mind's thinking power. Ever since I heard Yvonne's compelling story about the voice that she heard earlier in the morning and the message it carried, I've wondered: 'Why would red dots and a bruise be such a serious matter that the dreaded word "cancer" would even be considered as a causal factor for Samantha's symptoms?'. Throughout our lives, we've all had skin blemishes and spots on our skins, and while growing up, rambunctious me almost always had some form of bruise someplace on my body - picked up from rough play and goofing around with siblings in my native Jamaica. But cancer and skin lesions in the same sentence? This, I had not heard of before.

Wow, Cancer? What type of cancer causes red spots or bruises? Clearly, I had no competence to begin to answer these questions or to even understand why these could be cancer-related symptoms. I only wished Yvonne had more detailed answers to these questions from the 'voice'!

As a teenager, I came to understand some of the devastating effects of cancer on the human body: my mother developed breast cancer and appeared to have been cancer-free for several years. However, she died on March 15, 1979, after this monster of a disease reared its ugly head again and separated her from our lives. With all these historical thoughts swirling in my head, coupled with the reality of the moment, I couldn't imagine that this initial assessment of Samantha's underlying condition was accurate. To help my mental state cope with whatever was lying ahead, I thought I must make the admission to myself that whether the diagnosis would be validated, I am, and we are, going to do everything to help find ways through the medical system to make Samantha whole again.

We stopped and pulled into what looked like another "kiss and ride" area below the large emergency sign. There might have been signs on the wall stating that the area is only for drop-off and limited short-term parking. So, all three of us quickly came out of the minivan and walked through the emergency doors.

With the second letter in hand, we walked up to the front desk and told the male nurse on duty that we came from the Mississauga Trillium Hospital and were directed by Dr. Taylor to The SickKids Hospital. "The letter will describe more details," I said. He took the letter, read it, and asked for the customary health card, address, name of parent, etc. We were then asked to sit in the waiting area. Before sitting, I asked him for directions to the parking area, and he obliged.

I used this opportunity to leave Yvonne and Samantha in the emergency waiting area, and I drove to the parking garage at 100 Elm Street. As seen in the map below, this was another right turn off Elizabeth Street. Within a couple of minutes, I was at the entrance, where I pushed the button to get a parking ticket, drove into the underground garage, and was relieved to find a parking spot close to the elevators.

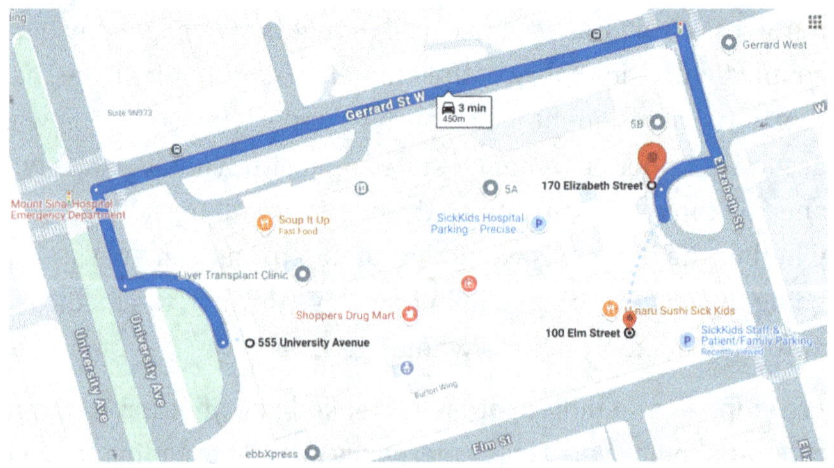

Source: https://www.google.com/maps

I hurried to the elevator and quickly pressed the button to take me up to the ground floor, where I followed the instructions and made a right turn, walked past the coffee shop on the left, then took the next left turn into the hallway, walked through a doorway and was back in the waiting room of the emergency area where Yvonne and Samantha were still sitting.

Within a few minutes, we were called to the front desk, given some brightly colored hospital registration forms, and told to make our way upstairs (to the 6th floor, we believe). We reversed the direction that I had just traveled to make our way to the elevator and pushed the button to the 6th floor. Again, we exited the elevator and followed the signs to navigate our way to the intake desk on the 6th floor, where we presented the colored forms to the attendant at the welcoming desk.

By now, we were sure that we had figured out the routine; surely, we would be asked to wait. Not this time around, however. Seeing that Dr. Taylor of Mississauga Trillium Hospital had called the SickKids Hospital ahead of our arrival, the receptionist at the front desk was expecting us. She rushed us into a room with a few pieces of furniture - only a bed and a single chair. She told us to place Samantha on the bed, and just then, a male doctor entered the room, introduced himself, went over to the bed, and started to examine the red spots and the bruises on Samantha's body. He asked a few questions; the most memorable being when we first spotted the bruises. He said that they needed to do blood work- a CBC- so that they could get to know more of what's happening. There was that acronym again, CBC. We ignored whatever CBC meant because, at this stage, we could sense that everyone was dealing with Samantha with some sense of urgency. He left the room, and within minutes, a female nurse came in with a small tray of vials and needles. For some reason we were observing everything, every movement, every body language, every conversation, spurred on likely by the sense of urgency with which the clinicians were going about their duties that were related to our young child.

The nurse took out the elastic band and asked us to have Samantha sit up on the bed. She examined Samantha's arms, and then she wrapped the elastic band around one of her arms. As she did that, we got the feeling that Samantha was not as scared as she was earlier in the day when blood was taken from her at Mississauga Trillium Hospital.

Within minutes, we would learn that those feelings were indeed true. The nurse explained to her that she might feel a small pinch and that she needed to do it because she had to take some blood. "Look away", she gently said to Samantha. As the needle pierced Samantha's arm, she remained calm and indifferent. This was very different from her reaction earlier in the day at Mississauga's Trillium Hospital when blood was being taken. On her second blood-giving experience, she might have reasoned that it was for her own benefit, or was it that she would have preferred not to be put into the stirrups? It was such a pity that she was too young to articulate her thoughts to us. Or, perhaps if she tried, we adults wouldn't understand.

*** The Beginning of Hospitalizations ***

The nurse took several vials of blood as was done at the previous hospital. She said, "You were good," to Samantha, and while leaving the room, she told us that the doctor would get the results shortly. About half an hour later, the same doctor who examined Samantha earlier entered the room. "We have the blood results", he said. He explained that the CBC showed that most of her cell lines were significantly reduced. At that moment, we didn't fully understand what that meant, but it didn't sound good to us.

He explained that immediate action was needed, and the next step was for her to receive two units of single-donor platelet transfusion because her platelet count was at a critically reduced level. He went on to explain that she had to be admitted into the hospital and observed for the next twelve hours and that another evaluation of her CBC would need to be done the next morning to determine the outcome of the transfusion on her platelet count.

Whew! That was quite a bit of information to unpack. Single donor! Platelet! Transfusion! Like most people, the term blood transfusion is one that we've heard before. Indeed, Cleveland's own mother had several blood transfusions in the 1970s. But, in this context, the term single-donor was new. Equally new was the term platelet. And why did a low platelet count seem to matter so much that it warranted immediate attention? Combined, all of this seemed confusing.

And then, she needed to be admitted! What could be so serious, we thought. Is it really Cancer? For us, Samantha's admission into the hospital called for an admission from both of us that Yvonne's encounter with the voice earlier that day was indeed as real as it could get. Something clearly spurred her to get our child to embark on the initial journey to the family doctor, then to the first hospital, and finally to the second hospital to which she is now admitted.

We needed to provide consent on behalf of Samantha so that the transfusion could be started. We didn't even deliberate to weigh the pros and cons.

We gave consent.

*** The Call Home ***

While on our way to SickKids, we had already called home to let Pauline know that we were on our way to the second hospital. We realized we now will need to let her know that Samantha is being admitted. So, while the staff made the necessary preparations, we called home and delivered the news about the continuously winding evolution of the day's journey. Samantha has been admitted to SickKids, Yvonne is spending the night with her, and Cleveland will be home sometime later in the night. This development shows that it's good to have a family to pick up the pieces when life happens. Grandma was able to provide dinner and the bedtime routine for the two children at home while their parents dealt with the decisions and uncertainties regarding the third child in a hospital that they had not planned to be in that night.

*** The Transfusion ***

The preparations for the transfusion were completed. The nurse who took the blood came into the room with what we understand to be the infusion pump and a drip bag attached to the intravenous (IV) pole on wheels. We thought that the color of the liquid in the bag would have been as red as blood, but the bag of liquid had a slightly cloudy-pale yellowish color. But Cleveland, not being the type of person who is shy to ask questions that to the learned seems dumb, said to the nurse, "I thought that the liquid for the transfusion would have been red, like blood, but why isn't it red?". She explained that this is not whole blood; it is just a part of the blood. Only the platelets are in the bag, and this does not include the red blood cells. That was satisfactory to us because we didn't know much about biology, but we were eager to learn what was going on with Samantha. At this moment in time, as this day went on, we realized that it was never too late to learn something new.

We didn't know it at the time, but we were in the early stages of continuous learning. We learned from the answers to questions about test results, explanations regarding medical terminologies, investigative processes, and the numerous conversations with staff. For reasons still unknown to us, on the night of May 15, 2003, Cleveland chose to start documenting as much as possible - conversations with the medical staff, blood work results, blood pressure, temperature, and almost every other bit of information that came our way.

We still have these scraps of paper with notes scribbled on them in our possession. Throughout the book, we will share some of them from the two binders worth of information that we collected. The collection started at SickKids on May 15, 2003, and continued until June 2024.

The following morning, Friday, May 16th, Cleveland called a dear work colleague with whom he has an excellent relationship to this day. Cleveland was booked to travel for work to Vancouver for a week starting the following Monday through to Friday. This was for a week-long training conference at which he was speaking each day. The conference center was booked, breakfast, lunch, and refreshments were arranged, and organizations had already committed their employees to attend. His presentations were completed and polished.

However, with all of what happened on Thursday the 15th, he knew that he was not traveling to Vancouver the following Monday. He updated her on the developments and suggested that they go ahead with the conference by asking a colleague from the corporate vendor that they represented to conduct the sessions. Rebecca was most understanding, and after he emailed her his presentation decks, she took hold of the entire event and executed the changes with his replacement, Emanuel. As Cleveland would later learn, they did it flawlessly. It's great when organizations hire good people, and Rebecca and Emanuel were two of the best, as good as any and better than many. Evidence of this is that Rebecca would later move on to run the Canadian division of a major multi-national technology corporation.

As you will later realize, Cleveland was away from work the following week.

*** Platelet Counts Matter ***

From the following image, we can see that Samantha's platelet count, when she was admitted on May 15, 2003, was two. From what we later learned in the summer of 2004 from my sister, who practices family medicine in the United States, and another physician in Canada, patients whose platelet counts are in the single digits (below ten) usually die within twenty-four to forty-eight hours, due to internal bleeding from vital organs. We were told that patients with platelet counts this low were usually referred to as having Severe Aplastic Anemia. Later still, we came to understand that the terminology was changed to Severe Acute Aplastic Anemia for patients whose platelet counts dropped to two or lower. No matter the nomenclature or scientific terms that were used, it was clear to us that low platelet counts were bad signals for her long-term health.

```
   7CX  -6886            THE HOSPITAL FOR SICK CHILDREN                PAGE 001
2003-05-17  17:28              (QNOLKP-014-054- MMPG)
                          DISCHARGE ORDER/SUMMARY

   STANBERRY, SAMANTHA                          HSC#:   2100777
   DOB: 2001-03-22                              WEIGHT(KG): 13.17
   ADMIT DATE: 2003-05-15                       UNIT: 7C
   SERVICE: PAEDIATRIC MED. PHONE: 416-813-6903 ADMIT#:  I3001842
   HSC RESPONSIBLE PHYSICIAN: PEER, MICHAEL MD
   HSC CONTACT: NOT AVAIL.                       PHONE: NOT AVAIL.


   DISCHARGE TODAY (2003-05-17), (MMPG)


   ALLERGIES:
      MED ALLERGIES
         2003-05-16    NO MEDICATION ALLERGIES KNOWN
      DIET ALLERGIES
         2003-05-16    NO FOOD ALLERGIES KNOWN


   MOST RESPONSIBLE DIAGNOSIS:
      PANCYTOPENIA

   OTHER DIAGNOSIS:
      SICKLE CELL TRAIT

   DISCHARGE MEDICATIONS:
      NO DISCHARGE MEDICATIONS

   DIET:
      USUAL DIET

   HOSPITAL COURSE/INVESTIGATION RESULTS:
      SAMANTHA IS A 2 YR OLD FEMALE WHO WAS ADMITTED MAY 15/03 WITH
   A 1 WEEK HISTORY OF BRUISING AND PETECHIAE. BLOODWORK ON ADMISSION
   SHOWED WBC 1.4, HGB 92, PLT 2 WITH BLOOD FILM SHOWING HYPOCHROMIA
   AND MICROCYTOSIS WITH NO BLASTS. RETICULOCYTE COUNT WAS 1.55%.
   PATIENT RECEIVED A PLATELET TRANSFUSION ON ADMISSION AND HAD A BONE
   MARROW BIOPSY THE FOLLOWING DAY.
      BONE MARROW ASPIRATE WAS HYPOCELLULAR WITH ALL 3 CELL LINES
   REDUCED. NO LEUKEMIC CELLS WERE SEEN.
      HEMATOLOGY HAS BEEN CLOSELY INVOLVED WITH PATIENT DURING THIS
   ADMISSION, AND AGREES WITH PLAN TO DISCHARGE HOME WITH DAILY CBCS
   TO BE DONE IN ER. PATIENT HAS FOLLOW UP ARRANGED WITH DR. KERBY ON
   WED MAY 21 AT HSC.
      PATIENT IS DISCHARGED HOME AFEBRILE, WITH VITAL SIGNS STABLE,
   AND NO ACTIVE BLEEDING.
      ON DISCHARGE MAY 17/03 CBC SHOWED WBC 1.5, HGB 84, PLATELETS
   18.

                          CONTINUED


===============================================================================
   STANBERRY, SAMANTHA YVONNE  2100777          DISCHARGE ORDER/SUMMARY
```


D → Hematology Clinic

If that is indeed the expected reality regarding the effect of single-digit platelet count on the human body, then if we had waited past Thursday the 15th until Saturday the 17th to visit the pediatrician (more than 48 hours after admission to SickKids), it is likely that Samantha would have died because of internal bleeding, caused by low platelet count.

If we were to hypothetically rewind the events of Thursday, May 15th, and imagine the future up to Saturday, May 17th, assuming that Samantha had not been admitted to SickKids hospital, then the alternate ending on Saturday, May 17th, might be that Samantha passed from this life to the next.

What would have been written as the cause of death on the death certificate? Internal bleeding due to low platelet count? Over the years, our entire family has pondered these thoughts and the implications that would have resulted if Yvonne had not taken matters into her own hands and left home to see the family doctor who triggered the sequence of events. We've always come back to the admission of gratefulness that Yvonne was obedient to the 'voice.' We collectively owe her a debt of gratitude!

* The Beginnings of Bone Marrow Aspirate Investigations *

The previous report copy is from the actual SickKids discharge form. It shows that Samantha was admitted on May 15, 2003, and discharged on May 17, 2003. It mentions that a bone marrow investigation was done to understand why some of her cell lines were reduced. The bone marrow investigation meant that she had to be anesthetized.

We were satisfied that they allowed us to be in the room with her while the anesthesiologist told her to count to ten while he squeezed the propofol into the port in her arm. How did we know it was propofol? We mentioned earlier that Cleveland was inquisitive. He asked questions about everything and took copious notes. A copy of the very first piece of paper on which these notes were taken is depicted below:

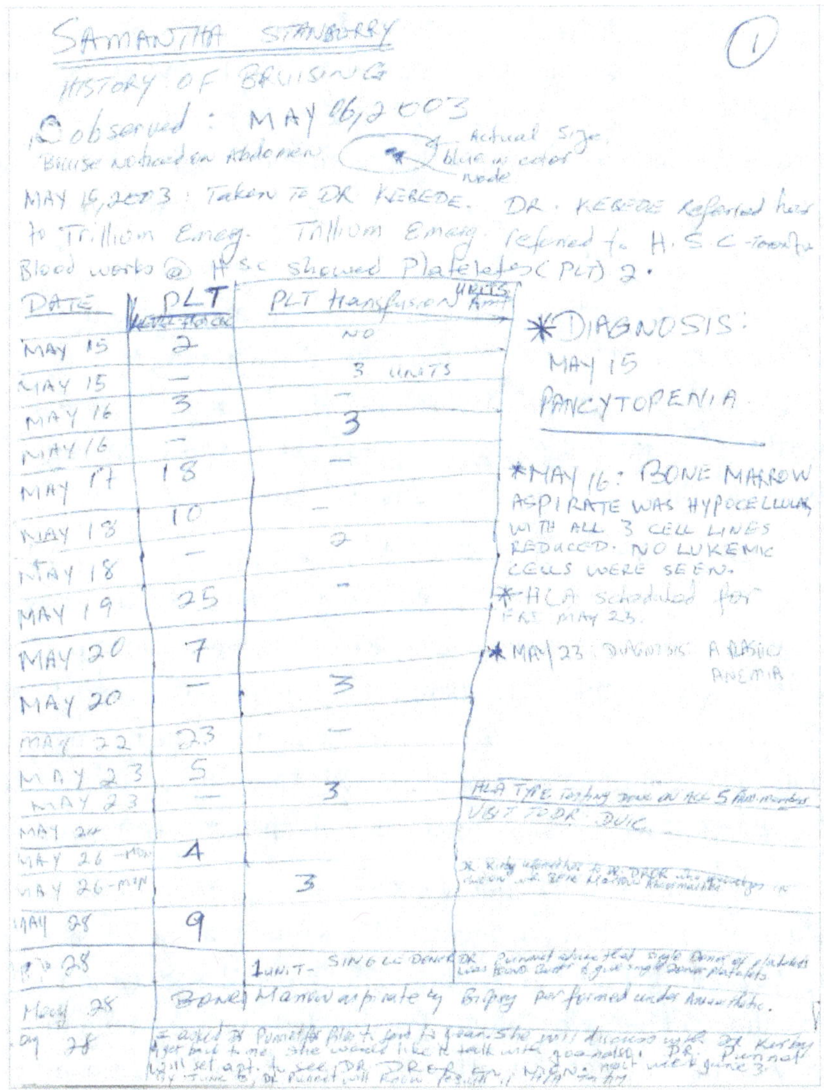

SAMANTHA STANBURRY (1)

HISTORY OF BRUISING

observed: MAY 16, 2003
Bruise noticed on Abdomen. [drawing] Actual Size. blue in color. node.

MAY 16, 2003: Taken to DR. KEBEDE. DR. KEBEDE referred her to Trillium Emerg. Trillium Emerg. referred to H.S.C - Toronto. Blood works @ HSC showed Platelets (PLT) 2.

DATE	PLT	PLT Transfusion (units Amt)
MAY 15	2	NO
MAY 15	–	3 UNITS
MAY 16	3	–
MAY 16	–	3
MAY 17	18	–
MAY 18	10	–
MAY 18	–	2
MAY 19	25	–
MAY 20	7	
MAY 20	–	3
MAY 22	23	–
MAY 23	5	
MAY 23	–	3
MAY 24		
MAY 26 - Mon	4	
MAY 26 - Mon		3
MAY 28	9	
MAY 28		1 UNIT - SINGLE DONOR
MAY 28	Bone Marrow aspirate by biopsy performed under Anaesthetic.	

*DIAGNOSIS:
MAY 15
PANCYTOPENIA

*MAY 16: BONE MARROW ASPIRATE WAS HYPOCELLULAR, WITH ALL 3 CELL LINES REDUCED. NO LUKEMIC CELLS WERE SEEN.

*HLA scheduled for FRI MAY 23.

*MAY 23: DIAGNOSIS: APLASTIC ANEMIA

HLA TYPE testing done on ALL 5 Fam. members
VISIT TO DR. DUIC

It is the collection of these notes and copies of medical records provided to us during this ordeal from 2003 to 2024 that enabled us to accurately write many parts of this book.

As seen in the scribbles above, her platelet count at admission on May 15th was 2. After she received two units of single-donor platelets, the platelet count dropped to 3 the following day, on May 16th. One doctor quipped, "What could be eating up her platelets so much?". We took that as an encouraging sign that the doctor was invested in trying to figure out the answer to her own rhetorical question.

She was given another platelet transfusion, and the platelet count went up to 18 at the time of her discharge on May 17, 2003. Yeah! Things were improving! At this time, we were getting very hopeful, so any bit of good news was encouraging. But were these encouraging signs about to last?

We were told to return to SickKids daily for the next four days - May 18th, 19th, and 20th- for blood work, and on Wednesday, May 21, to see the Oncologist, Dr. Kirby. So, we traveled back and forth from and to the hospital over those days. Some days, Cleveland alone went with Samantha while Yvonne managed the home front. It didn't remain this way for long, however. We had to figure out what was going to be the long-term arrangements.

One decision we made that week is one that we are proud to stand by to this day. We decided that Samantha's sickness, however long it might last, should not affect the education and livelihood of her two siblings. We decided that we would find a way for her siblings to continue to attend school and any other usual activities as they normally would do as much as possible.

The discharge form showed exactly what we wanted to see and what we were verbally told, "NO LEUKEMIC CELLS WERE SEEN." This meant that she doesn't have Leukemia! She does not have cancer! Another piece of good news. But then again, was this good news?

Over the next four days and beyond, we would come to understand that the most important metric being measured and tracked to keep Samanta alive was the platelet count. She could get a transfusion, and the count would go up to 18, 10, or 25, only to drop to the single digits again.

The graph below shows the see-sawing of the platelet counts from the first eight days of May 15, 2003 (platelet counts on the left and the collection dates at the bottom). Every single spike up to counts of 10, 18, 25, or even 7 were after receiving platelet transfusions a day prior. This information is visualized from the CBC bloodwork records provided to us by the SickKids Hospital.

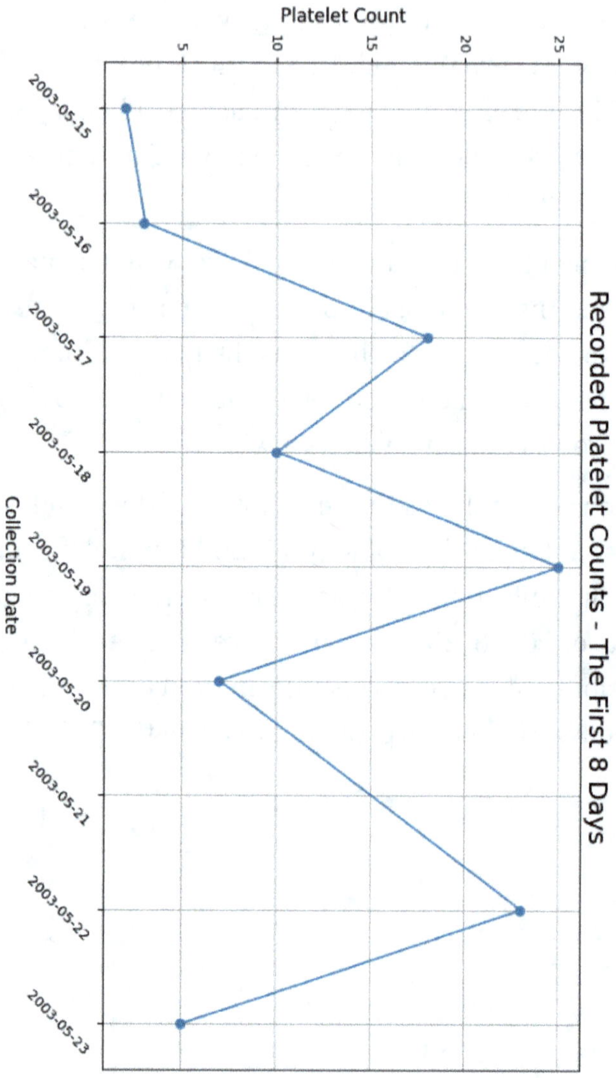

Platelet Count
Recorded Platelet Counts - The First 8 Days
Collection Date
5
10
15
20
25
2003-05-15
2003-05-16
2003-05-17
2003-05-18
2003-05-19
2003-05-20
2003-05-21
2003-05-22
2003-05-23

3

The Diagnosis

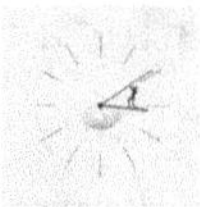

Because platelet count was, without exception, the number one metric that was always at the top of the list of items discussed since we arrived at the SickKids Hospital, it became clear to us that platelet count is the value to watch. But what are platelets anyway? One of the early days in the week of May 19th, while holding Samantha in his arms, Cleveland, being the inquisitive person he is, asked this question of the oncologist. Below is a gist of the conversation:

Cleveland: "Dr. Kirby, what are platelets?"

Dr. Kirby: "Platelets are cells in our body that allow our blood to clot so that when we have a cut, we don't bleed continuously".

Cleveland: "So what is causing hers to drop so much?"

Dr. Kirby: "We are not sure at the moment. We know that it's not leukemia; that's cancer. The bone marrow aspirate allowed us to rule that out".

Cleveland: "Oh, so that's good, that it's not cancer!".

Dr. Kirby: "No, that's not good. We know how to treat cancer, but we now believe that the problem is caused by Aplastic Anemia, and we don't exactly have the formula to treat it as much as we know how to treat leukemia".

Here comes another new term.

"Aplastic Anemia?" Cleveland whispered.

Dr. Kirby: "Aplastic Anemia is usually caused when the long bones are not making good cells. These bones are usually the leg bones. Since we know that after a transfusion of platelets on day one, the count drops dramatically on day two, we know that her bone marrow is not making them properly. Think of the bone marrow as a factory that makes different types of chairs. Some chairs are red, and some are platelet chairs. In her case, the factory is making good red chairs, but it's not making good platelet chairs. The treatment is different from cancer in the sense that we now must go into the factory and stop it from making defective platelet chairs. In her case, the factory is the bone marrow, and the platelet chairs are just platelets. We need the bone marrow to start making good platelets".

Cleveland: "I understand the explanation. So, what do we do next?".

Dr. Kirby: "We want to do an HLA-type testing of your family to find out if any of you are a match for a bone marrow transplant. We would like to schedule for your family to do the testing on Friday May 23rd."

Cleveland: "And, what does that test for? Is it blood type? Samantha and I have the same blood type, so does that mean I will be a match?".

Dr. Kirby: "The HLA testing will determine more than blood type. It will determine if any of you are a good HLA match, including other things beyond blood type. We could then schedule that person and Samantha to come into SickKids, and we would take the bone marrow from that donor and transfer it to Samantha. Once the test is done, you would also be placed on a global bone marrow registry, and if you are a match to anyone else, you could be asked if you're willing to donate your bone marrow". She provided us with an appointment sheet - a copy of the actual sheet is shown below:

Samantha Stanberry

HLA TYPING

On _May 23/03_ HLA typing, a blood test, has been arranged for your family. Please go to room 408 main floor, Ambulatory Diagnostics (beside Shoppers Drug Mart) to register. **(It opens at 730am, but please register <u>no later than 9am.</u>)** It is not necessary to go to outpatient registration as the necessary information will have been provided for pre-registration to have been completed. Be sure that each family member has their health card with them on that day. The phone number for Ambulatory Diagnostics is 813- 5913

Now that the HLA test date was settled, uncertainties abound, so the conversation continued.

Cleveland: "So, what causes Aplastic Anemia?".

Dr. Kirby: "We really don't know the cause. We do know that it is very rare. It affects about 3 people in a population of 1 million each year. Because we will be treating her for Aplastic Anemia, I will be transferring her treatment to Dr. Dror, who works in that area of hematology and would be better able to determine the best course of treatment".

The initial thought after the first blood tests at SickKids was that the diagnosis was Pancytopenia. This term was also new to us, but we later learned that this is a disease condition that causes low levels of red blood cells, white blood cells, and platelets. Even though her initial CBC results reflected low levels of all three lines, the diagnosis was changed from Pancytopenia to Aplastic Anemia. The figures below show CBC results for May 20th and May 22nd.

```
                    The Hospital for Sick Children
                Department of Paediatric Laboratory Medicine

Patient:          STANBERRY,SAMANTHA YVONNE                   DOB:    2001-03-22
 SC#:             2100777                                     Sex:    F
 Location:        Emergency                                   Reg #:  E3004002
Responsible MD:  DR.Carole O'Beirne

        Autosend Report (NOT a Chart Report) printed 2003-05-20 at 12:46h

  T25948    COLL: 2003/05/20 11:50 REC: 2003/05/20 12:03 PHYS: Scolnik,Dennis

       CBC
          WBC              C 1.4           (5.0-12.0)     X 10^9/L
          RBC              L 3.25          (4.00-5.00)    X 10^12/L
          HGB              L 82            (110-140)      g/L
          HCT              L 0.247         (0.350-0.420)
          MCV              L 75.9          (80.0-94.0)    fL
          MCH                25.2          (24.0-31.0)    pg
          MCHC               332           (320-360)      g/L
          PLT              C 7             (150-400)      X 10^9/L
          MPV               .6.3           (4.0-14.0)     fL


             Department of Paediatric Laboratory Medicine
       Phone: Core Laboratory 8800   Microbiology 6000   Blood Bank 6208

Patient:          STANBERRY,SAMANTHA YVONNE                   DOB:    2001-03-22
 HSC#:            2100777                                     Sex:    F
 Location:        Haematology Service Clinic                 Reg #:  A3017046
Responsible MD:  Kirby,Melanie
            Autosend Report (NOT a Chart Report) printed 2003-05-22 at 0907h

  H37824    COLL: 2003/05/22 08:39 REC: 2003/05/22 08:41 PHYS: Kirby,Melanie

                                                                          STAT
       CBC
          WBC              C 1.5           (5.0-12.0)     X 10^9/L
          RBC              L 3.42          (4.00-5.00)    X 10^12/L
          HGB              L 87            (110-140)      g/L
          HCT              L 0.256         (0.350-0.420)
          MCV              L 74.7          (80.0-94.0)    fL
          MCH                25.6          (24.0-31.0)    pg
          MCHC               342           (320-360)      g/L
          PLT              PENDING
          MPV              PENDING
          CBC Comment      PENDING
```

A few days later, we were given additional information from SickKids explaining Aplastic Anemia. Below is a copy of parts of the information from the hand-out that we received. This information would later help to inform us on the course of treatment options that we were given.

- AA-MDS-TALK Mailing List
- The Aplastic Anaemia Trust
- The Myelodysplastic Syndromes Foundation

Anemia-Related Links

- PNH On-Line Support Group
- Fanconi Canada
- Anemia Institute for Research and Education
- Thalassemia Foundation of Canada
- The Sickle Cell Association of Ontario
- Lupus Canada
- Canadian Celiac Association

Blood-Related Links

- Canadian Blood Services
- Hema-Quebec
- Bone Marrow Registry
- CIMFR - Canadian Inherited Marrow Failure Registry
- National Blood Safety Council
- Canadian Hemophilia Society

What are Aplastic Anemia and Myelodysplasia?

Aplastic anemia is a rare but extremely serious disorder that results when the marrow fails to produce blood cells. Aplastic anemia may be either acquired or inherited.

Myelodysplasia is similar to aplastic anemia in that production of blood cells is decreased; however, the blood cells which are produced in myelodysplasia may not function properly. Aplastic anemia patients who do not receive a bone marrow transplant may go on to develop myelodysplasia which, in turn, can progress to leukemia.

How Common?

Aplastic anemia is a rare disease. It is estimated that there are 2 to 12 new cases per million population per year. It occurs in both adults and children. Myelodysplasia is more common, with the majority of patients being over the age of 50.

The Function of Bone Marrow

The central portion of bones is filled with a spongy red tissue called bone marrow. The bone marrow is essentially a factory producing the cells of the blood: red cells that carry oxygen from the lungs to all areas of the body; white cells that fight infection by attacking and destroying germs, and platelet cells (platelets) that control bleeding by forming blood clots in areas of injury. Continuous production of blood cells is necessary all through life because each cell has a finite life span once it leaves the bone marrow and enters the blood:

- red cells: 120 days;
- platelets: 8 - 10 days;
- white cells: one day or less.

Healthy bone marrow is a superb blood cell factory and supplies as many cells as needed, increasing production of red cells and platelets when bleeding occurs and of white cells when infection threatens.

When bone marrow cell production fails, normal levels of red cells, white cells, and platelets begin to fail. Bruising, bleeding, infection, tiredness, pallor, and other symptoms of anemia may develop.

What Causes Aplastic Anemia and Myelodysplasia?

Although a congenital chromosomal abnormality may predispose one to develop inherited aplastic anemia, the medical community does not know the cause of most cases of acquired aplastic anemia. Certain toxic chemicals, medications, viral infections and radiation exposure appear to cause both myelodysplasia and aplastic anemia, but millions of people with exposure to the same factors do not develop either disease.

How are Aplastic Anemia and Myelodysplasia Treated?

Treatment depends upon the patient's age, the severity of the disease, and the availability of an HLA-matched donor.

Supportive Care

- **Blood Transfusions**
  Red cells and platelets from volunteer donors can temporarily correct some of the cell deficiencies. Unfortunately, resistance to platelets usually develops, and long-term use of red cell transfusions can lead to a condition known as iron overload.
- **Prevention and Treatment of Infection**
  Infection is a great danger to patients due to the depletion of white cells. Broad-spectrum antibiotics are often used liberally.
- **Emotional and Psychological Support**
  Patients with aplastic anemia and myelodysplasia require a great deal of emotional support to help them deal with the implications of these serious disorders. Upon diagnosis, patients and their family members may feel lost in a maze of unfamiliar medical terminology and puzzled about the diagnosis of a disease which they may never have heard of. The Aplastic Anemia Association of Canada can explain the diseases in terms the layperson can understand. Many patients require assistance in adapting to the chronic health concerns and life restrictions imposed by the diagnosis. Both patients and their family and friends often become discouraged when therapies are slow or unsuccessful. Volunteers with personal experience with the disease are happy to provide valuable guidance and support during these times of need.

Medical Treatment Options

http://www.aamac.ualberta.ca/   5/25/2003

Aplastic Anemia and Myelodysplasia Association of Canada   Page 4 of 5

1. **Aplastic Anemia**

   o **Bone Marrow Transplantation**
      Bone marrow transplantation is the treatment of choice for patients with severe aplastic anemia who are under 50 years of age and who have an HLA-identical sibling donor. Long-term survival rates for these patients are 80% or better.
   o **Hematopoietic Stimulation (Bone Marrow Stimulation)**
      Aplastic anemia patients who are not candidates for bone marrow transplantation may be given drugs such as anabolic steroids and/or hematopoietic growth factors (GM-CSF, G-CSF and IL-3) to stimulate their own bone marrow to improve blood production.
   o **Immunosuppression**
      Non-transplanted aplastic anemia patients may also receive drugs such as ATG, ALG, methylprednisolone and cyclosporine. These drugs appear to prevent the body's own attack on its bone marrow: by suppressing the patient's immune system, the disease process is sometimes reversed.

2. **Myelodysplasia**
   Although some myelodysplasia patients have responded to experimental drug therapies, bone marrow transplantation remains the only cure for the disease.

How Can You Help Aplastic Anemia and Myelodysplasia Patients?

You can help by doing the following:

- Donate blood and platelets for transfusions
- Sign up with the Unrelated Bone Marrow Registry
- Volunteer with the Aplastic Anemia Association of Canada
- Give generously to the Aplastic Anemia Association of Canada

The Association

Mandate

- Inform the public about Aplastic Anemia and Myelodysplasia
- Provide a nation-wide support network for patients, families and medical professionals
- Support Canadian Blood Services blood programs and the Unrelated Bone Marrow Registry
- Raise funds for medical research

We completed the day's visit after the platelet transfusion. When she was not hospitalized, platelet transfusions were either done in the emergency department or in a room at the eighth-floor hematology clinic called the "Day Care." The daycare was staffed by superbly capable and competent practitioners who knew their craft well. We still remember Rita, who could locate the veins needed to transfer platelets from bag to body with expert precision.

May 23rd came, and we all traveled to SickKids for the HLA appointment. With arms extended, we all gave, and the nurses received blood. "Give, and you shall receive," Cleveland quipped. But we were doing the giving, and the nurse was doing the receiving. This was, however, for a potential lifesaving cause, especially with Cleveland crossing his fingers tightly that he would be a match. He had previously blurted out, "I am confident that I will be a match because Samantha and I share the same blood type." These moments helped to provide some level of relief and hid the stresses that we felt.

Fast forward to the results of the HLA-type testing, which came back sometime in early September 2003, and despite Cleveland's hope and confidence that he would be a match, the results stated that no suitable marrow donor had been found in our immediate family. However, hope was not lost; the hospital had access to millions of individuals from hundreds of countries so that they could search for a match. Below is a copy of page one of the letter received explaining this to us.

The Diagnosis

The Hospital for Sick Children -- Bone Marrow Transplant Program

Search Process for an Unrelated Donor

Tissue typing (HLA typing) has been completed on your immediate family and no suitable marrow donor has been found. The following outlines the search procedure used to identify an unrelated donor.

We have computer access to approximately 8 million individuals from about 20 countries (50 registries) who have agreed to be registered as potential donors. Searches are done by national registries. A world wide summary of donors is available which directs us to the registries with the best chance of having a donor for your child (Cord Blood registries are searched). This search process is coordinated through the Canadian Blood Services, Unrelated Bone Marrow Donor Registry (UBMDR) in Ottawa. Your child's HLA type along with a search request is forwarded to the UBMDR as soon as a decision is made to look for an unrelated donor. The Canadian UBMDR is always searched first. However, when necessary, multiple registries can be searched at the same time.

Each individual has 6 HLA antigens (2 markers for each of A, B, DR) on their white blood cells. An ideal match is a 6 of 6 match using testing done by detailed chemical methods (molecular typing). Occasionally minor degrees of mismatch are acceptable. Many of the antigens can be divided into subgroups. Most donors are listed on the registries with only the A and B antigens reported and without specific subgroups. Therefore, the first identification of a potential donor is a 4 of 4 match using broad typing (no subgroups). The next step is to upgrade the typing to determine DR and identify any subgroups (specific typing). To do this, batches of potential donors are contacted by their National Registry and requested to give a blood sample for further testing which is done in their own city. If a 6 of 6 match is identified, another blood sample is requested which is then sent to Toronto for confirmatory testing, which includes molecular testing. Donors are often excluded at this last step. It may be necessary to test several hundred individuals to find a matched donor. When a suitable donor is identified, your Haematologist/Oncologist will be notified at once. The average time to identify a donor is 3 to 4 months.

A request to "activate" a donor is faxed to the Canadian UBMDR. The potential donor will be notified by the marrow collection centre in their city, and called in for an information session to explain how marrow is harvested and the possible risks to the donor. The donor is requested to consent to the procedure. Following this, the donor has a complete medical examination. Occasionally donors are eliminated for medical reasons. A detailed screen for infectious disease is done on the marrow donor just like the screen done on regular blood donors. Only then is the donor confirmed and a harvest scheduled. From identifying a donor to obtaining marrow usually takes 1 to 2 months. Once the donor is confirmed, you and your child will have a consultation with one of the transplant physicians to discuss the transplant.

<u>Other Important Information</u>
1. The search process is confidential. Neither your child nor potential donors are identified in any way.

Coming back to May 23rd, 2003, during the next week, we searched on the internet for information regarding Aplastic Anemia and went to a local library to find books on the disease. However, limited information was available. I phoned my physician sister and asked why there's not much information, and she said that it's such a rare disease that little research and information is known about it. I would later learn that some medical students might not have even been taught about it in their university program.

While speaking with some parents, we learned that they initially had to convince healthcare workers and law enforcement that they did not abuse their children with a blunt instrument. As seen above in the hand-out that we received, only about 2 to 12 cases per 1 million in the population are diagnosed each year. In the year 2003, Samantha would have been one of those 3 or 12 people out of a population of one million who was diagnosed with Aplastic Anemia.

4

The Treatment

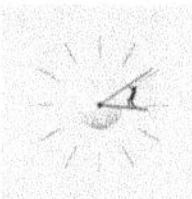

We were introduced on our next clinic appointment, to Dr. Dror. However, before that, we went through our now-accustomed registration process. The registration desk was conveniently located beside the entrance door on floor 8 at the hematology clinic, on the left side of the elevator. The front-line staff at this clinic were super nice, even though they were doing emotional labor, registering and attending to adults who were at some of their lowest and saddest moments in life. They treated every single parent and guardian with dignity.

After registration, we would be instructed to get blood drawn from a vein in the arm or a 'finger-poke.' The blood collection queue is against a wall opposite the registration desk. For almost ten years, it was the same nurse, Connie, who did the finger poke or took the blood. She was the nicest blood-taker that the clinic could have. Her demeanor remained first-class and wonderfully caring throughout our almost decade-long interaction with her. Samantha would normally just look at her quietly without saying a word as she either takes blood from a vein or uses a device to prick one or more fingers and then extract blood for analysis.

The clinic also had a pleasant patient liaison who would come into the well-laid-out waiting area, decked out with a playground with which the very sick children could interact. She would get to know the parents and provide information on seminars that parents could attend to learn more about the various diseases that their children were battling. She would provide information on parent support groups that are available. She would also pair up parents who wanted to provide support with parents who needed support. Yvonne was paired up with a parent-supporter, and later, she also supported other parents by sharing some of what she did to aid in the management of her child.

Children with several diseases were treated in this clinic. They include Myelodysplasia, Leukemia, and Aplastic Anemia, among others. Despite the reality that these dangerous illnesses were being managed by this clinic, the environment was a strange dichotomy of sad and worried-looking parents surrounded by pleasant staff, including front-desk registration staff, nurses, patient liaison offices, doctors, and a child–friendly, playful environment.

This environment created a distraction for both the children and especially the worried parents. Parents sometimes engage in playing games with the children. Children at this clinic ranged in age from months-old babies to about seventeen years old.

Play in the waiting area would often be interrupted by an announcement over the clinic's intercom, such as "Samantha Stanberry to the blue room." Once we heard that, we knew that it's our queue to go to one of the waiting rooms in the color that was just announced.

It was in one of those rooms where we met Dr. Dror on May 26th, 2003. He would be managing the treatment for the recently diagnosed Aplastic Anemia. Dr. Dror was a quiet-speaking person. He introduced himself and described Aplastic Anemia. He gave us some options for treatment per below:

A. Bone Marrow Transplant

B. Immune System Suppression

Option A was not immediately possible because we had given the blood samples only the Friday before.

Option B treatment primarily included an experimental cocktail of drugs that, while proved effective in animal investigations, were not conclusive in humans.

We could sense that there was an urgency to provide treatment above and beyond platelet transfusions. Cleveland asked him, "What is the probability of recovering from this without using the drug cocktail or without using platelet transfusion?".

The response was bleak but somehow provided clarity regarding the decision to be made. Apparently, the results in the animal studies showed about 80% success with the drug cocktail and 20% failure (death) with transfusion only.

The decision was easy and clear. We signed onto the drug cocktail treatment.

***** Rabbit or Horse *****

The visualization below shows platelet counts recorded during the month of May 2003. The major takeaway is that in the month of May 2003, her platelets shot up to values such as 18 or 25, as seen on the 17th, and 19th respectively. These rises in platelet counts were all due to platelet transfusions. Indeed, by the end of May, the count was below 10.

Even though these results show about two weeks of platelet transfusion, we now believe that they highlight the reality that platelet transfusion was not a tenable treatment solution.

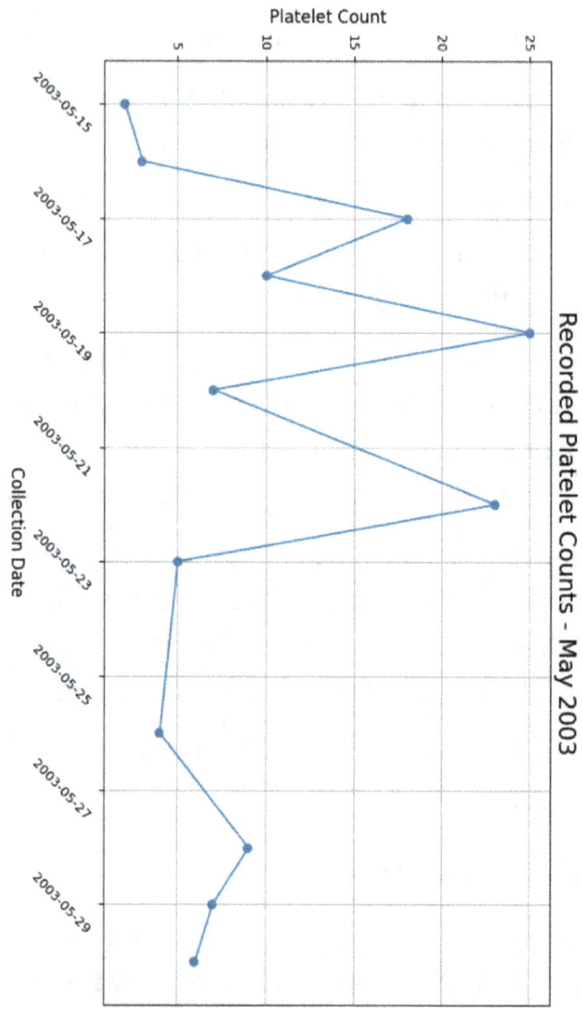

We agreed with Dr. Dror's recommendation to start the Immune System Suppression treatment. However, how is this done? Can medical science really prevent someone's immune system from functioning? So, what happens if her immune system is suppressed and she gets a cold, the flu, or is bitten by a mosquito? We would later discover answers to all these questions that were swirling around in our heads.

Dr. Dror explained in terms we could understand that the immune system is the army of cells and other systems that go to battle and fight foreign infections after they enter our bodies. In Aplastic Anemia, he explained, the platelets are not being made properly, so the immune system detects this and, therefore, tries to shut down the place or factory where these are being made. This is the reason why the immune system needs to be suppressed until the factory can be repaired.

To suppress, stop, or make the immune system work less, we were told that several drugs would need to be administered. Samantha would also need to be admitted for about a week. We decided to divide the responsibilities. One thing we decided is that Samantha would always have one of us in the hospital with her. Since Yvonne never liked driving on the highways, the decision was that Cleveland could travel between home and the hospital while Yvonne stayed with her during the hospitalization. Cleveland would visit daily during this week of treatment. Samantha and Yvonne were in the hospital from June 2, 2003, to June 8, 2003.

Some nurses are just awesome. Sometime on June 2, one of them saw the scribbles that Cleveland was making on paper, and we think she must have felt sorry for him and told him that we have journals that you can use to make your notes. She provided us with printed copies of journal pages that we could use to capture the notes that we were taking. Whew! These nice pages were a calming wind! It seems that when one is under incredible stress, any bit of 'goodness' can be overwhelmingly heart-warming. We appreciated it so much.

This wonderful, nice nurse gave us copies of a journal to capture Samantha's journey. The nurse even completed the first page of the journal for us. The journal entry below, titled "ADMITTED TO 6C JUNE 2, 2003, TO START TREATMENT", is Cleveland's chicken scratch handwriting. The remaining sections were completed by the same nurse who gave us the journal. She gave us a kick start to document that family's journey, and thanks to her, we have copies to share today. Prints of some of these copies of the admission journal and discharge order summary are depicted below:

Sick Kids'
Family Journal

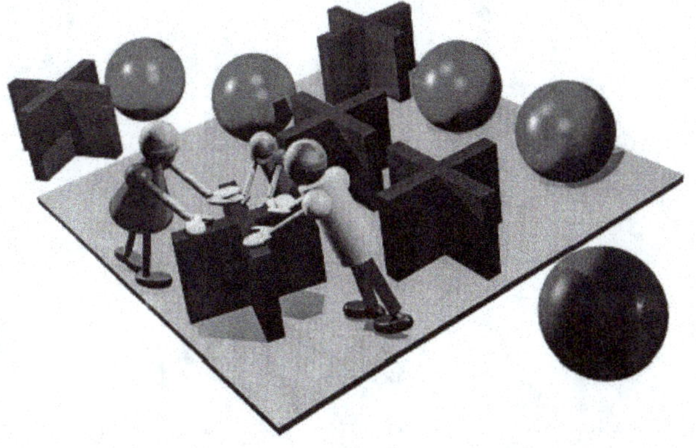

Working together – sharing all that we know

This Journal belongs to 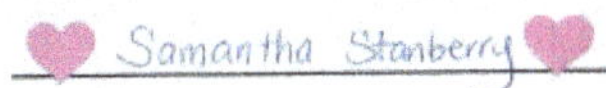 Samantha Stanberry

Over-the-counter Medications/Remedies

ADMITTED TO 6C JUNE 3 2003 TO START TREATMENT

Occasional Medicine and Complementary or Alternative Remedies (i.e. Tylenol, Vitamins, Cough Syrup, Echinecea etc.)

Name and strength of medicine/ remedy	Did someone recommend the medicine? If yes, who? (Name and Specialty)	What is the medicine for?	Amount given at each dose	Number of times given every day	Comments (how your child takes it, reactions etc.)	Start Date	Finish Date
Cyclosporin	Dr. Yigal Dror (Haem)	Stimulate white blood cell production (helps fight infection)	80mg.	Twice/day.	ADMITTED TO H.S.C	June 2 2003	
Pentamidine IV	Dr. Yigal Dror	antibiotic that prevents pneumonia	55mg	once every two weeks		June 3 2003	
Platelets CMV⊖ irradiated	Dr. Yigal Dror	low platelets level 14.	2 units	She will get platelets when level below 30.	no reaction.	June 3 2003 p.m.	
Prednisone .	Dr. Yigal Dror	steroid to help her body deal with stress + infection.	14mg.	Twice/day.	Stop it slowly take it with food or milk/juice watch her urine output	June 4 2003 a.m.	
Platelets CMV⊖ irradiated	Dr. Yigal Dror	low platelets level 22.	2 units	Once only.		June 4 2003	
ATGAM	Dr. Yigal Dror	blood products of immune globulins that will ↑ her wbc	550mg.	Once daily 4x in a row.	Given over 8 hrs. High risk of reaction so we give it slowly + benadryl + tylenol	June 4 2003	
Diphenhydramine (Benedryl)	Dr. Yigal Dror	antihistamine to prevent allergic reactions	13mg IV	before each dose of ATGAM + in emergency/allergic reaction	Makes Samantha hyper then sleepy.	June 4 2003	
Acetaminophen (tylenol)	15am Dr. Yigal Dror	Pain / fever	150mg	before each dose of ATGAM and in case of fever		June 4 2003	
Meperidine (Demerol)	Dr. Yigal Dror	Extreme Pain + spasms	13mg IV	Only if she has ↑pain and spasms with ATGAM.	not given yet given @ 6:30pm.		

*Medications come in different strengths. Please include the strength of your child's medication when filling in this chart. For example: 1 teaspoon of Tylenol 80 milligrams per milliliter is different than 1 teaspoon of Tylenol 160 milligrams per milliliter

Sick Kids' Family Journal

Prescribed Medications

Medicine Ordered By Health Care Professional

*Name and strength of medicine	Who prescribed the medicine? Name and Specialty	What is the medicine for?	Amount given at each dose	Number of times given every day	Comments (how your child takes it, reactions etc.)	Start Date	Finish Date
Niphedipine	Dr. Yigal Dror	to decrease high blood pressures.	2.0 mg.	Only given if BP is above 110/70 (maximum 4 times)	not given yet	June 4/03	
Gentamicin		fight infection Antibiotic	35 mg	once		June 4/03 @12pm	
Tazocin		Antibiotic				June 5/03 1pm?	
Gentamicin IV		Antibiotic	35mg			June 5/03. 9:05Am.	
Platelets		Low platelets				June 5/03 12:15am.	
cmv ⊕		level 25	½ unit				
T·ILENOL		Prevention of fever	2ml			June 5 4:05pm	
?		Reduce blood pressure ft. 133/40		when needed		June 5 5:00pm	
~~Prednisone~~ Dr. 14mg = 2·8ml		~~Stool softener~~ ~~14mg - 280ml~~				~~June 5~~ 9:00pm	
LACTULOSE		STOOL SOFTENER	3335mg 5 ml			JUNE5 9:00 P.m	
Ranitidine IV		Reduce upset stomach (vomiting)	15mg .			June 5/02 11:20 pm	
Amlodipine		Reduce blood Pressure	3mL .	once-bedtime		June 7/03 @ 9:30pm	

*Medications often have more than one name. Include all the names you know.
Medications come in different strengths. Please include the strength of your child's medication when filling in this chart. For example: 1 teaspoon of Tylenol 80 milligrams per milliliter is different than 1 teaspoon of Tylenol 160 milligrams per milliliter

```
6CX  -6551          THE HOSPITAL FOR SICK CHILDREN
2003-06-08  15:57            (QNOLKP-009-007- MMSK)           PAGE 001
                          DISCHARGE ORDER/SUMMARY

STANBERRY, SAMANTHA                          HSC#:  2100777
DOB: 2001-03-22                              WEIGHT(KG): 14
ADMIT DATE: 2003-06-02                       UNIT: 6C
SERVICE: NEUROLOGY        PHONE: 416-813-6911 ADMIT#:  I3002476
HSC RESPONSIBLE PHYSICIAN: HITZLER, HANS MD
HSC CONTACT: NOT AVAIL.                       PHONE: NOT AVAIL.
________________________________________________________________


DISCHARGE IN PM OF TODAY (2003-06-08), (MMAG)


ALLERGIES:
   MED ALLERGIES
      2003-05-16   NO MEDICATION ALLERGIES KNOWN
   DIET ALLERGIES
      2003-05-16   NO FOOD ALLERGIES KNOWN
________________________________________________________________

DISCHARGE CONTINGENT UPON:
DISCHARGE CONTINGENT UPON: DRINKING WELL
DISCHARGE CONTINGENT UPON: EATING NORMALLY
DISCHARGE CONTINGENT UPON: PAIN MANAGED
DISCHARGE CONTINGENT UPON: VITAL SIGNS STABLE
DISCHARGE CONTINGENT UPON: TEMPERATURE NORMAL.
MD TO SEE PATIENT PRIOR TO DISCHARGE
DISCHARGE CONTINGENT UPON --AFEBRILE AND CULTURES NEGATIVE

MOST RESPONSIBLE DIAGNOSIS:
APLASTIC ANEMIA

OTHER DIAGNOSIS:
FEBRILE NEUTROPENIA

DISCHARGE MEDICATIONS:
AMLODIPINE 2.5 MG BY MOUTH DAILY BEFORE BED FOR 14 DAYS
RANITIDINE INJ 15 MG BY MOUTH 2TIMES DAILY FOR 10 DAYS
CYCLOSPORINE NEORAL 70 MG BY MOUTH 2TIMES DAILY FOR 30 DAYS

DIET:
USUAL DIET

HOSPITAL COURSE/INVESTIGATION RESULTS:
   28 YRS OLD GIRL W APLASTIC ANEMIA ADMITTED TO START RX.(ATG AND
CSA).TOLERATED RX. WELL W NO PROBLEMS.HAD 4 DOSES OF ATG
     HER CSA LEVEL INITIALLY IS 215 AND DOSE REDUCED TO 70 MG Q 12
HR.TARGET LEVEL IS 150 TO 200.LEVEL WILL BE CHECKED BEFOR
DISCARGE.SHE DEVELOPED F/N.CULTURES NEGATIVE.COVERED WITH
ANTIBIOTICS FOR 72 HOURS

                        CONTINUED

================================================================
STANBERRY, SAMANTHA YVONNE  2100777          DISCHARGE ORDER/SUMMARY
```

From memory and from the records that we kept, we believe that the drugs that we were told would be used to suppress the immune system are the following:

Atgam

Cyclosporine

Pentamidine

Atgam, we were told, is harvested from either Rabbits or Horses. Her dose of Atgam was derived from Horses. The Atgam was given over a period of eight hours. Other medications and platelets were given, as indicated in copies of the family journal above. As seen in the copy of the discharge form above, SickKids was comfortable with discharging her for home care because she was drinking well, eating normally, and had stable vital signs and a normal temperature.

Additionally, we were given prescriptions for additional drugs to be taken at home following her discharge. These were:

1. Cyclosporin

2. Prednisone

3. Ranitidine

4. Amlodipine

Each of the above medications came with their own unique schedule. We now had a challenge of ensuring that the correct dose of medication was given at its prescribed time, such as giving her before or after a meal, or the volume to be given.

In some cases, such as with Cyclosporin and Prednisone, the medication had to be tapered. Meaning that the first five doses might be 2.8 mL while the next three should be 2 mL, the next three should be 1.5 mL, and for the next five only 1 mL should be given. This was the case with Prednisone.

There is no way we could easily manage this from memory or by only reading the instruction labels attached to the medication containers. To aid us, SickKids gave us a calendar for all the drugs, along with a taper schedule.

As shown below are copies of the calendar and taper schedule that we first used starting on June 9, 2003. June 18th at 8:00 PM was the last date that Ranitidine was given.

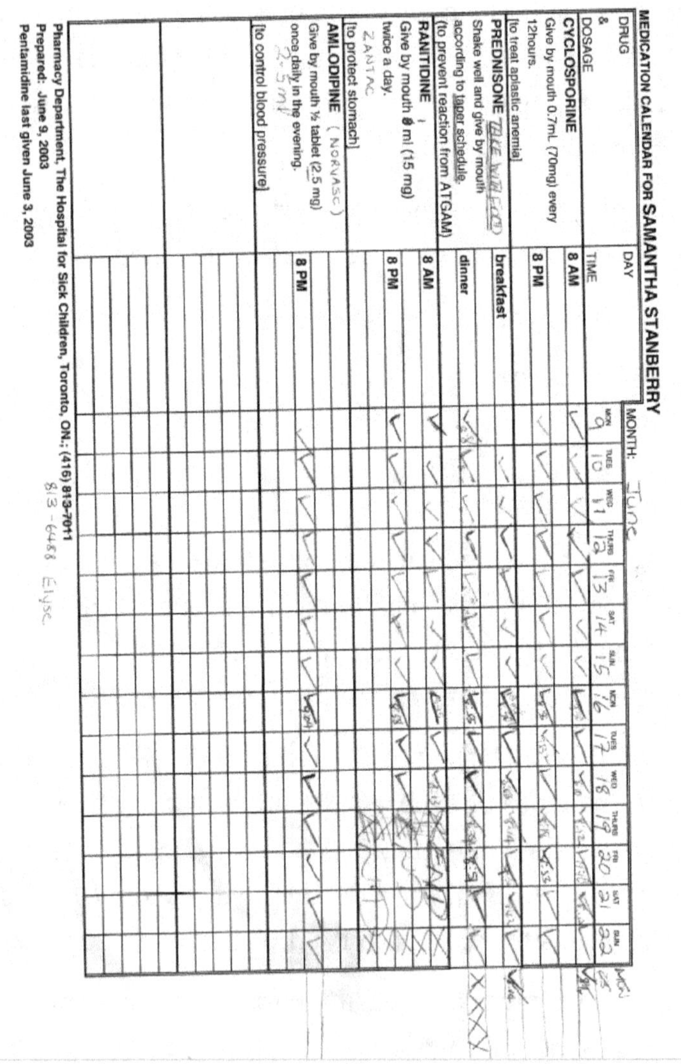

MEDICATION CALENDAR FOR SAMANTHA STANBERRY

MONTH: June

DRUG & DOSAGE	DAY / TIME	MON 9	TUES 10	WED 11	THURS 12	FRI 13	SAT 14	SUN 15	MON 16	TUES 17	WED 18	THURS 19	FRI 20	SAT 21	SUN 22	MON 23
CYCLOSPORINE Give by mouth 0.7mL (70mg) every 12hours. [to treat aplastic anemia]	8 AM															
	8 PM															
PREDNISONE TAKE WITH FOOD Shake well and give by mouth according to taper schedule. (to prevent reaction from ATGAM)	breakfast															
	dinner															
RANITIDINE Give by mouth 8 ml (15 mg) twice a day. ZANTAC [to protect stomach]	8 AM															
	8 PM															
AMLODIPINE (NORVASC) Give by mouth ½ tablet (2.5 mg) once daily in the evening. 2.5ml [to control blood pressure]	8 PM															

Pharmacy Department, The Hospital for Sick Children, Toronto, ON.; (416) 813-7011
Prepared: June 9, 2003
Pentamidine last given June 3, 2003

Prednisone Taper for SAMANTHA STANBERRY — STARTED Prednisone June 9th (mon)

DATE	breakfast dose	dinner dose
until June ~~13~~th	~~14 mg (2.8 mL)~~	~~14 mg (2.8 mL)~~
June 14, 15 & ~~16~~	~~10 mg (2 mL)~~	~~10 mg (2 mL)~~
June 17, ~~18~~ & ~~19~~	7.5 mg (1.5 mL)	~~7.5 mg (1.5 mL)~~
June 20, ~~21~~ & ~~22~~	~~5 mg (1 mL)~~	~~5 mg (1 mL)~~
June ~~23~~, ~~24~~, 25 & 26	5 mg (1 mL)	NONE
June 27th	STOP	

Prepared: June 9, 2003
The Hospital for Sick Children, Department of Pharmacy

The chart below shows that Prednisone's last dosage was on Wednesday, June 25, 2003. Amlodipine's last dosage was a day earlier at 8:07 PM on June 24th.

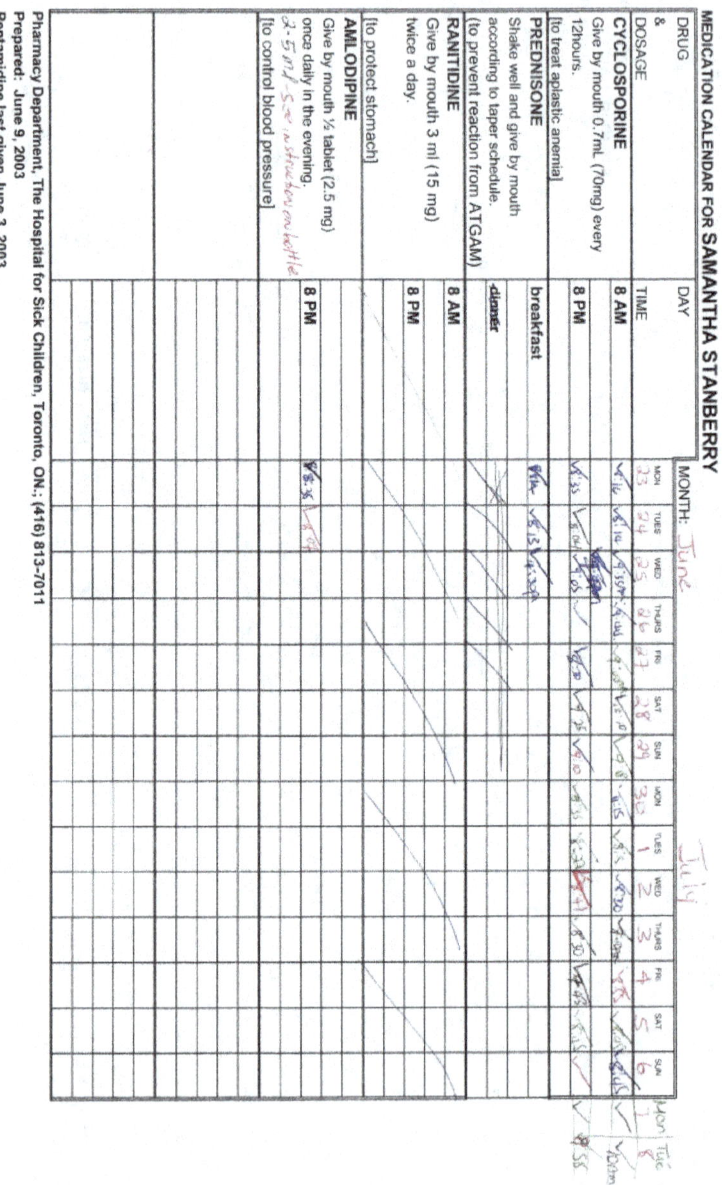

MEDICATION CALENDAR FOR SAMANTHA STANBERRY

MONTH: June / July

DRUG & DOSAGE	DAY / TIME	MON 23	TUES 24	WED 25	THURS 26	FRI 27	SAT 28	SUN 29	MON 30	TUES 1	WED 2	THURS 3	FRI 4	SAT 5	SUN 6	Mon 7	Tue 8
CYCLOSPORINE Give by mouth 0.7mL (70mg) every 12hours. [to treat aplastic anemia]	8 AM	✓8:16	✓8:14	✓9:35	✓9:00	✓9:00	✓8:10	✓9:00	8:15	✓8:15	✓8:20	✓7:00	✓8:5	✓8:45	✓	✓	✓
	8 PM	✓8:35	✓8:04	✓9:05		✓8:30	✓9:25	✓9:10	✓8:35	✓8:30	✓	✓8:30	✓8:45	✓8:15	✓		✓8:55
PREDNISONE Shake well and give by mouth according to taper schedule. (to prevent reaction from ATGAM)	breakfast	✓na	✓8:13	✓4:30?													
	~~dinner~~																
RANITIDINE Give by mouth 3 ml (15 mg) twice a day. [to protect stomach]	8 AM																
	8 PM																
AMLODIPINE Give by mouth ½ tablet (2.5 mg) once daily in the evening. 2.5ml - see instruction on bottle [to control blood pressure]	8 PM	✓8:35	✓8:04														

Pharmacy Department, The Hospital for Sick Children, Toronto, ON.; (416) 813-7011
Prepared: June 9, 2003
Pentamidine last given June 3, 2003

The medication chart was kept fastened to the fridge with a magnet and as we looked at it on June 25th, we had some sense of achievement that we could cross off the milestones that we had met. We could now focus on giving Samantha the last remaining medication at the top of the list below:

1. Cyclosporin
2. Prednisone
3. Ranitidine
4. Amlodipine

We thought that Cyclosporin alone would continue to be given for the remainder of her treatment. The medication calendar below up to July 20th proved that we understood what was going on and were correct.

MEDICATION CALENDAR FOR SAMANTHA STANBERRY

DRUG & DOSAGE	DAY / TIME	MON 7	TUES 8	WED 9	THURS 10	FRI 11	SAT 12	SUN 13	MON 14	TUES 15	WED 16	THURS 17	FRI 18	SAT 19	SUN 20
	MONTH: July														
CYCLOSPORINE Give by mouth 0.7mL (70mg) every 12hours. [to treat aplastic anemia]	8 AM	✓	✓	✓	✓	✓	✓	✓	✓	✓	✓	✓	✓	✓	✓
	8 PM	✓	✓	✓	✓	✓	✓	✓	✓	✓	✓	✓	✓	✓	✓
PREDNISONE Shake well and give by mouth according to taper schedule. (to prevent reaction from ATGAM)	breakfast														
	dinner														
RANITIDINE Give by mouth 3 ml (15 mg) twice a day. [to protect stomach]	8 AM														
	8 PM														
AMLODIPINE Give by mouth ½ tablet (2.5 mg) once daily in the evening. [to control blood pressure]	8 PM														

Pharmacy Department, The Hospital for Sick Children, Toronto, ON.; (416) 813-7011
Prepared: June 9, 2003
Pentamidine last given June 3, 2003

We didn't understand fully what was going on. And neither were we correct for very long regarding a single medication. By July 21st, as seen in the chart below, another medication, Zovirax, was added to the list of life-saving drugs needed to save her from the ravages of Aplastic Anemia. Fortunately, this drug was only given for eight days.

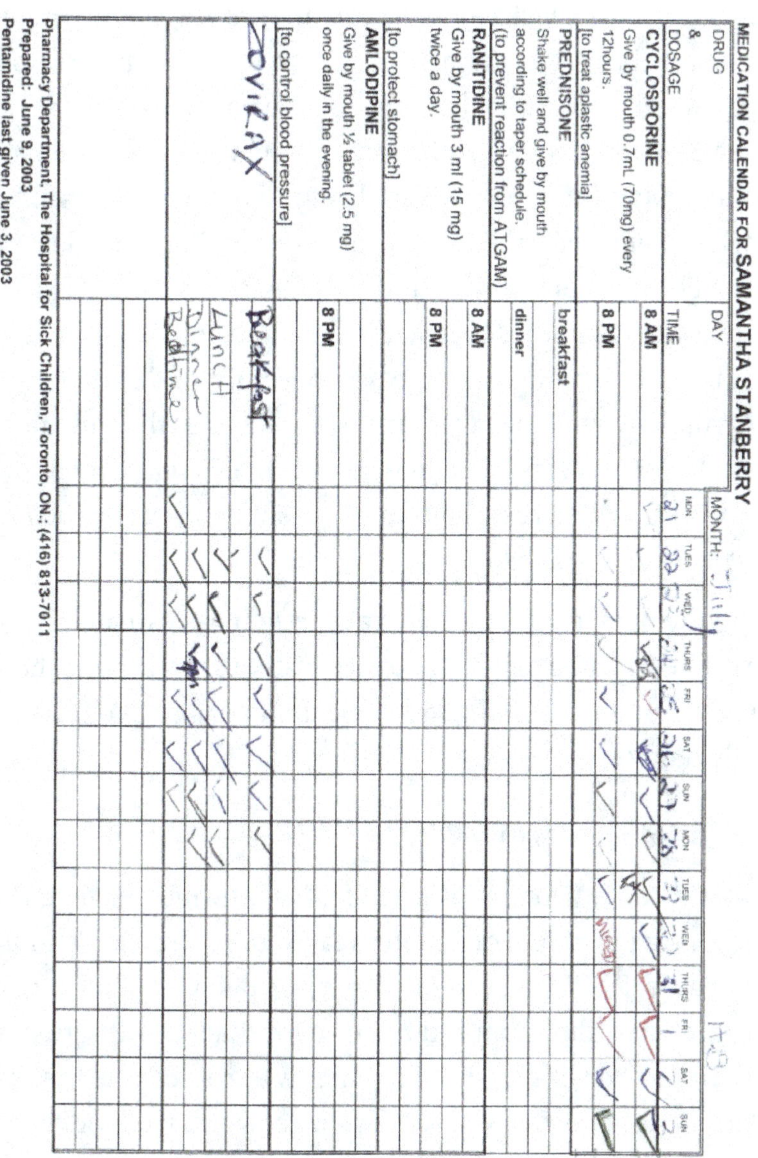

MEDICATION CALENDAR FOR **SAMANTHA STANBERRY**

MONTH: July

DRUG & DOSAGE	DAY / TIME	MON 21	TUES 22	WED 23	THURS 24	FRI 25	SAT 26	SUN 27	MON 28	TUES 29	WED 30	THURS 31	FRI 1	SAT 2	SUN 3
CYCLOSPORINE Give by mouth 0.7mL (70mg) every 12hours. [to treat aplastic anemia]	8 AM														
	8 PM														
PREDNISONE Shake well and give by mouth according to taper schedule. (to prevent reaction from ATGAM)	breakfast														
	dinner														
RANITIDINE Give by mouth 3 ml (15 mg) twice a day. [to protect stomach]	8 AM														
	8 PM														
AMLODIPINE Give by mouth ½ tablet (2.5 mg) once daily in the evening. [to control blood pressure]	8 PM														
ZOVIRAX	Breakfast														
	Lunch														
	Dinner														
	Bedtime														

Pharmacy Department, The Hospital for Sick Children, Toronto, ON.; (416) 813-7011
Prepared: June 9, 2003
Pentamidine last given June 3, 2003

So, how could we give her 0.7 mL of Cyclosporine or 1.0 mL of Ranitidine? Could we measure these medications in such precise quantities accurately? Well, the answers to those questions lie in the fact that the SickKids Hospital in Toronto, Ontario, Canada, is a globally best-in-class institution. We were given various sizes of syringes by the hospital that could easily measure the liquid from 3 mL to as small as 0.1 mL. Cleveland's days as a head boy studying the University of Cambridge's O Levels at Frankfield Comprehensive High School (now Edwin Allen High School) and A Levels at Excelsior Community College (both in Jamaica) came in extremely handy. My teachers would have been proud of me as I taught Yvonne to avoid parallax errors, and I tried my best to avoid any when we were measuring Samantha's medications. Parallax errors can creep in when the eye is positioned incorrectly when reading measurements on a scale, such as a test tube or syringe.

But why did we get so lucky that someone as capable as Yvonne could be at home every day to accurately give our daughter the medication by following the intricate tapering schedules in the early days?

*** The Single Income ***

In April 2002, Yvonne returned from maternity leave to her corporate job at one of Canada's large telecommunications providers. Pauline (Yvonne's mom) helped with childcare support, and she promised to do so for one year. It's great to have a mother like that! Seeing that we are a couple that usually plan, sometimes five years in advance, we started looking at what daycare costs would be a year away. We contacted many daycare centers to get their existing rates and figured that the cost might follow inflationary pressures and go up another two percent a year from April.

The reality was that daycare for two children and afterschool care for one child (our son would be in grade 1 in September 2003) would not make economic sense for our family. We decided in about May 2002 to start running a mock-budget using Cleveland's larger income as the sole family income and ignoring Yvonne's income completely – a pro forma budget. When we got married, we decided to have joint expenses and bank accounts, and this worked for our situation. As an aside, we still operate this way with that same bank account thirty-one years later!

This mock budget would ignore Yvonne's income so that we could have a realistic financial preview of how we would run the household if Yvonne were to resign from her corporate job. We ran this budget until March 2003. The mock budget proved that with some budget cuts, we could function. We were short a few months, but it was clear to us that we could function.

Armed with this observed information, in mid-April 2003, Yvonne submitted her resignation and gave two weeks' notice of her intentions to leave the organization. The firm asked her if she could stay on for another two weeks. Yvonne agreed to the request and ended her employment with the firm on Friday, May 9th, 2003.

During Yvonne's final week at the firm, the first spots were noticed on Samantha on May 6th, as seen at the top of the notes below. As Yvonne tried to enjoy her new-found freedom from corporate life, she spent much of Monday, May 12th, enjoying her time at home with her children. However, she used much time that day, telephoning the pediatrician to secure an appointment on Saturday May 17th, so that he could help with the spots on Samantha. By Monday the 12th, more spots were showing up. And by Thursday the 15th, we now know that Yvonne heard "the voice."

SAMANTHA STANBURRY ①
HISTORY OF BRUISING

Observed: MAY 06, 2003
Bruise noticed on abdomen — Actual size, blue in color. node.

MAY 15, 2003: Taken to DR. KEBEDE. DR. KEBEDE referred her to Trillium Emerg. Trillium Emerg. referred to H.S.C - Toronto. Blood works @ HSC showed Platelets (PLT) 2.

DATE	PLT	PLT Transfusion (Units/Amt)
MAY 15	2	NO
MAY 15	—	3 units
MAY 16	3	—
MAY 16	—	3
MAY 17	18	—
MAY 18	10	—
MAY 18	—	2
MAY 19	25	—
MAY 20	7	
MAY 20	—	3
MAY 22	23	—
MAY 23	5	—
MAY 23	—	3
MAY 24		
MAY 26 -thu	4	
MAY 26 -min		3
MAY 28	9	

* DIAGNOSIS:
MAY 15
PANCYTOPENIA

*MAY 16: BONE MARROW ASPIRATE WAS HYPOCELLULAR WITH ALL 3 CELL LINES REDUCED. NO LEUKEMIC CELLS WERE SEEN.
*HLA scheduled for FRI MAY 23.
* MAY 23 DIAGNOSIS: APLASTIC ANEMIA

HLA TYPE testing done on May 5 from members. VISIT TO DR. DUIC.

So, that's how it came to be that Yvonne was home to administer the series of medications. In hindsight, we either did not run the mock budget for almost a year to determine if we could afford to live on Cleveland's income nor did we do it to avoid paying daycare costs for three children.

We believe that unbeknownst to us, divine powers were looking out for us and helped to guide our thinking and decision-making. We can't imagine that, as excellent as daycare centers might be, they could accurately administer the various medications that Samanta needed to keep her alive. We believe that we were sent on the mock-budget exercise to arrive at the decision for Yvonne to quit her job so that she could be home to give Samantha the cocktail of drugs that she needed at the time and schedule that they should be given. But was this the only reason why Yvonne was now a stay-at-home mom? A week wouldn't go by before we got the answer in no uncertain terms.

The Severe Acute Respiratory Syndrome (SARS) outbreak in 2003 only added to our worries. With Samantha's immune system now severely compromised, we were advised to do everything to prevent her from getting an infection. We had to stop her from playing outdoors and would need to test her temperature daily. If her body temperature were above 38 degrees Celsius, we would need to take her to SickKids emergency.

A temperature above 38 degrees sent us to the hospital on many occasions. Some of these dates are May 19th, 20th, 29th, June 11th and 12th. The emergency discharge sheets below help to highlight these experiences.

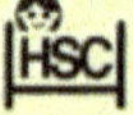

-02   **EMERX-8885**
(QEMRE3)

THE HOSPITAL FOR SICK CHILDREN

EMERGENCY VISIT DISCHARGE INFORMATION SHEET

STANBERRY, SAMANTHA YV
E3003872
2100777
2001-03-22
2003-05-19   09:43

Child's regular doctor: DUIC, ANDREW D.

Discharge diagnosis: Blair Inox

Your child has been assessed in the Emergency Department at The Hospital for Sick Children.
This is an emergency assessment and diagnosis only. As it is often difficult to recognize and treat
all aspects of any condition at a single visit, it is important that you follow the instructions listed below.

Instruction handouts given:

- ❑ Vomiting and Diarrhea
- ❑ Asthma / Wheezing
- ❑ Head injury
- ❑ Febrile Seizure
- ❑ Fever
- ❑ Croup
- ❑ Wound Care
- ❑ Cast Care
- ❑ Sedation
- ❑ Other:

Medications:

-
-
-

Other instructions:

Come to EC May 20/03 — (for
(per 25) monitors

- ❑ Follow up with your child's family doctor or paediatrician in __________ days, or sooner if necessary.
- ❑ A referral will be made to the __________________ clinic.
- ❑ Lab results pending: __________________   ❑ We will call (positive results only)
     ❑ Check results with family doctor

If your child's condition is not improving or is worsening, you should contact your child's regular doctor.
If you cannot reach your doctor, you may bring your child back to the Emergency Department,
or you can obtain free medical telephone advice from Telehealth Ontario at 1-866-797-0000.

Your signature below indicates that you understand the information on this sheet.

Instructions given by   Parent, guardian, or patient's signature

Date: __________   Time: __________   *White copy on chart*   *Yellow copy to patient*

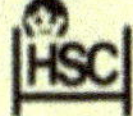

-02   (QEMRE3)   EMERX-9445

THE HOSPITAL FOR SICK CHILDREN

EMERGENCY VISIT DISCHARGE INFORMATION SHEET

STANBERRY, SAMANTHA YV
E3004002
2100777
2001-03-22
2003-05-20   11:38

Child's regular doctor: _DUIC, ANDREW D._

Discharge diagnosis: _low platelets — recovered 2 wout. plts_

Your child has been assessed in the Emergency Department at The Hospital for Sick Children. This is an emergency assessment and diagnosis only. As it is often difficult to recognize and treat all aspects of any condition at a single visit, it is important that you follow the instructions listed below.

Instruction handouts given:

❑ Vomiting and Diarrhea   ❑ Febrile Seizure   ❑ Wound Care   ❑ Other:
❑ Asthma / Wheezing   ❑ Fever   ❑ Cast Care
❑ Head injury   ❑ Croup   ❑ Sedation

Medications:

* _______________________________________
* _______________________________________
* _______________________________________

Other instructions:

[illegible handwriting]

[illegible handwriting]

❑ Follow up with your child's family doctor or paediatrician in __________ days, or sooner if necessary.

❑ A referral will be made to the ____________________ clinic.

❑ Lab results pending: ____________________
  ❑ We will call (positive results only)
  ❑ Check results with family doctor

If your child's condition is not improving or is worsening, you should contact your child's regular doctor. If you cannot reach your doctor, you may bring your child back to the Emergency Department, or you can obtain free medical telephone advice from Telehealth Ontario at 1-866-797-0000.

Your signature below indicates that you understand the information on this sheet.

____________________   ____________________
Instructions given by   Parent, guardian, or patient's signature

Date: ____________   Time: ________

White copy on chart   Yellow copy to patient

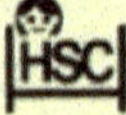

-02   **EMERX-3466**

(QEMRE3)

THE HOSPITAL FOR SICK CHILDREN

STANBERRY, SAMANTHA YV
E3004963
2100777
2001-03-22
2003-05-29   13:02

EMERGENCY VISIT DISCHARGE INFORMATION SHEET

Child's regular doctor: _DUIC, ANDREW D._

Discharge diagnosis: _Aplastic Anemia — Platelet transfusion_

Your child has been assessed in the Emergency Department at The Hospital for Sick Children.
This is an emergency assessment and diagnosis only. As it is often difficult to recognize and treat
all aspects of any condition at a single visit, it is important that you follow the instructions listed below.

Instruction handouts given:

❏ Vomiting and Diarrhea   ❏ Febrile Seizure   ❏ Wound Care   ❏ Other: _WBC 0.9_
❏ Asthma / Wheezing   ❏ Fever   ❏ Cast Care
❏ Head injury   ❏ Croup   ❏ Sedation   _Hemoglobin 74_

Medications:

- ____
- ____
- ____

Other instructions:

1) You need to come here immediately if she has a fever more than 38, if she has mucosy bleeding is weak or pale, or has cough
2) Follow up with Dr. Abby of primary recommended tomorrow

❏ Follow up with your child's family doctor or paediatrician in __________ days, or sooner if necessary.

❏ A referral will be made to the _______________________ clinic.

❏ Lab results pending: _______________________
     ❏ We will call (positive results only)
     ❏ Check results with family doctor

If your child's condition is not improving or is worsening, you should contact your child's regular doctor.
If you cannot reach your doctor, you may bring your child back to the Emergency Department,
or you can obtain free medical telephone advice from Telehealth Ontario at 1-866-797-0000.

Your signature below indicates that you understand the information on this sheet.

_______________________   _______________________
Instructions given by   Parent, guardian, or patient's signature

Date: _May 11/03_   Time: _1423h_

                            White copy on chart   Yellow copy to patient

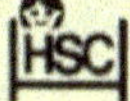

-02   **EMERX-9330**
(QEMRE3)

HSC   **THE HOSPITAL FOR SICK CHILDREN**

EMERGENCY VISIT DISCHARGE INFORMATION SHEET

STANBERRY, SAMANTHA YV
E3006326
2100777
2001-03-22
2003-06-11   22:33

Child's regular doctor: DUIC, ANDREW D.

Discharge diagnosis: _______________________

Your child has been assessed in the Emergency Department at The Hospital for Sick Children. This is an emergency assessment and diagnosis only. As it is often difficult to recognize and treat all aspects of any condition at a single visit, it is important that you follow the instructions listed below.

Instruction handouts given:

❑ Vomiting and Diarrhea   ❑ Febrile Seizure   ❑ Wound Care   ❑ Other:
❑ Asthma / Wheezing   ❑ Fever   ❑ Cast Care
❑ Head injury   ❑ Croup   ❑ Sedation

Medications:

• _______________________
• _______________________
• _______________________

Other instructions:

____
____
____
____
____
____

❑ Follow up with your child's family doctor or paediatrician in __________ days, or sooner if necessary.
❑ A referral will be made to the _______________________ clinic.
❑ Lab results pending: _______________________   ❑ We will call (positive results only)
  ❑ Check results with family doctor

If your child's condition is not improving or is worsening, you should contact your child's regular doctor. If you cannot reach your doctor, you may bring your child back to the Emergency Department, or you can obtain free medical telephone advice from Telehealth Ontario at 1-866-797-0000.

Your signature below indicates that you understand the information on this sheet.

_______________________   _______________________
Instructions given by   Parent, guardian, or patient's signature

Date: _______________   Time: _____________   White copy on chart   Yellow copy to patient

THE HOSPITAL FOR SICK CHILDREN

Ambulatory Patient SARS Screening Tool

1. Fill out sections A, B and C:

SECTION A:

- Have you had unprotected contact with a person with SARS in the last 10 days? ☐No — ☐Yes ⇐ Quarantine applies; notify Public Health
- In the last 10 days have you been to a health care facility that has been closed due to SARS? ☐No — ☐Yes ⇐ Quarantine applies; notify Public Health
- Are you under quarantine, or have you been contacted by public health and put on home isolation? ☐No — ☐Yes ⇐ Quarantine applies; notify Public Health

In the last 10 days, have you been to any other health care facility (i.e. hospital, rehabilitation centre, long-term care facility)? ☐No ☐Yes

If "yes", list the facility(s) ________________

SECTION B:

Have you returned from a SARS affected area in the last 10 days? ☐No ☐Yes

SECTION C:

Are you experiencing **any** of the following symptoms [worse than usual]?

Myalgia (muscle aches)
Malaise (severe fatigue)
Severe headache
Shortness of breath
Cough
Fever

lethargy/irritability (younger children)
difficulty breathing (younger children)
loss of appetite (younger children)

☐No ☐Yes ⇐ Record temperature ____ °C

⇐ Is temperature at or above 38°C? ☐No ⇐ PASS ☐Yes ⇐ FAIL

2. SCREENING RESULT [to be completed by screener]:

- ☑ PASS If NO to A and B and C
- ☐ PASS If YES to only B [provide educational materials]
- ☐ PASS If YES to only C with no fever
- ☐ FAIL If YES to A ⇐ Quarantine applies; Public health to be notified.
- ☐ FAIL If YES to C PLUS fever ⇐ give [VISITOR/ CHILD] a mask and direct to outpatient setting
- ☐ FAIL If YES to B + C regardless of fever ⇐ give person a mask and direct to Adult Emergency Department [call ahead] or to HSC Emergency if a child

Screener Name (Please Print):	Signature:		Date:
Michael Camus			June 12/03
Interviewee Name (Please Print):	Phone #:	Signature:	Date:
Stanberry Samantha Yvonne	510 - 1234	Stanberry	June 12/03

HSC Revised May 20, 2003 — CHART COPY — 35351/ G123

We think that the graphical representation in the following calendars better describes what needed to be done and why Yvonne truly needed to be free from the responsibilities of corporate duties, as we engaged with this disease previously unknown to us.

MAY 2003

SUN	MON	TUES	WED	THURS	FRI	SAT
27	28	29	30	1	2	3
4	5	6 • Red dots observed	7 • Red dots remain	8 • Red dots remain	9 • Bruise observed. Red dots remain. Yvonne's last day at firm	10 • Bruise remain. Even more red dots appear
11	12 • Yvonne's 1st day as stay-at-home-mom • Appointment secured with pediatrician	13 • Bruise remain. Even more red dots appear	14 • Bruise and red dots remain	15 • The voice. • Family Dr. trip • Hospitals 1 & 2 trips (Sick Kids) • Platelet transfusion given • Hospitalization	16 • Platelet transfusion given • Hospitalized	17 • Platelet transfusion given • Discharged from Sick Kids
18 • Bruise remain. More red dots appear. • Sick Kids trip • Blood works done • Platelet transfusion given	19 • Sick Kids trip • Blood works done	20 • Sick Kids trip • Blood works done • Platelet transfusion given	21 • Sick Kids trip • Appointment with Oncologist • Blood works done	22 • Sick Kids trip • Blood works done • Platelet transfusion given	23 • Sick Kids trip • Family had HLA testing • Blood works done • Platelet transfusion given	24 • Examine bruises and if new ones found - get to Sick Kids within one hour
25 • Examine bruises and if new ones found - get to Sick Kids within one hour	26 • New bruise found • Sick Kids trip • Blood works done • Platelet transfusion given	27 • Examine bruises and if new ones found - get to Sick Kids within one hour	28 • New bruise found • Sick Kids trip • Blood works done • Platelet transfusion given	29 • New bruise found • Sick Kids trip • Blood works done • Platelet transfusion given	30 • New bruise found • Sick Kids trip • Blood works done • Platelet transfusion given	31 • Examine bruises and if new ones found - get to Sick Kids within one hour

Yvonne needed to be available to travel back and forth between SickKids while Cleveland figured out how to keep the remaining two children's lives stable. In the last two full weeks of May 2003, she would be at SickKids every day except for about four days.

The following month of June 2003 would kick off as a similarly busy month for both Yvonne and Samantha. Samantha was admitted on June 2 to start the immune suppression treatment. As agreed, Yvonne would spend each day and night at her bedside, even for the eight-hour-long Atgam infusion. Yvonne would later recall how difficult it was for her to leave Samantha's side to get coffee or a snack downstairs. However, let's not get too sad here. Help was on the way.

"A friend will love and care for you at all times" is a paraphrase of a quote from one of the wisest people to ever live. And lucky or blessed or fortunate for Yvonne, she had such a friend. They met at the firm from which she had just recently resigned and continued their friendship. This stalwart of a human being, Pamela, was effectively retired from work, and she would pop up at just the right times.

"Pamella just showed up minutes after I called her to tell her that I was in the hospital with Samantha," Yvonne would recall. Pamella lived within fifteen to twenty minutes' walk from Sick Kids. "Go ahead and take a break, girl. Have some coffee or tea and walk around. I'm here and will take care of everything", Pamela would say in her always bubbly manner. Samantha was already familiar with Pamela, so these caused no alarm for her. During this second hospital stay, Pamela was a constant presence at Samantha's side.

The calendar below captures the hospital stays and other daily happenings during the month of June far better than they could be described using only words.

JUNE 2003

SUN	MON	TUES	WED	THURS	FRI	SAT
1 • Examine bruises and if new ones found - get to Sick Kids within one hour	2	3	4 • Hospitalized • Immune Suppression treatment begins • Platelet transfusion as required	5	6	7
8 • Discharged from Sick Kids • Take medications at home	9 • Sick Kids trip • Blood works done	10	11 • Sick Kids trip • Blood works done	12 • Sick Kids trip • Blood works done	13	14
15	16 • Sick Kids trip • Blood works done • Platelet transfusion	17	18	19	20 • Sick Kids trip • Blood works done • Platelet transfusion	21
22	23	24	25 • Sick Kids trip • Blood works done • Platelet transfusion	26	27	28
29	30 • Sick Kids trip • Blood works done					

The month of June 2003 would have been particularly testing for Yvonne. By June, Cleveland was back at work, bringing in the single household income. He would need to use a single vehicle to drive to work, so this meant that at times, for each way of the journey, Yvonne needed to travel for two hours from home in Mississauga to SickKids in Toronto by taking public transportation. She would need to take two buses and two Toronto Transit System subway rides. She would reverse this route to get back home. On one such occasion, Yvonne recalled how she struggled to get the stroller with Samantha sitting in it up the steps of the subway and onto University Avenue. "I was so tired and struggling with the stroller", she reminisced. "Two ladies appeared out of nowhere, one helped with the stroller and the other carried the toddler's bag up the set of stairs" Yvonne recalled.

By the end of June 2003, we were planning to keep the regular weekly appointments at the clinic. However, we were instructed to examine Samantha's head and body every day. If any spots or bruises were found, or her temperature was above 38 degrees Celsius, we should take no longer than one hour to get to either the hematology clinic on the 8th floor during day-light hours, Monday to Friday, or to the emergency department at other times. These daily examinations resulted in us going to SickKids almost daily for two or three weeks, then every other day, then twice per week, weekly, then monthly. Each visit to the clinic would result in a platelet transfusion. Each visit to the emergency department also resulted in a platelet transfusion.

The months from July 2003 to November 2003 continued to be samples of June 2003. We could write about each day of each month in detail. However, since we have the CBC records along with platelet transfusions, we are of the opinion that to save pages of paper, we would share the information in the following charts.

Suffice it to mention, however, that when Cleveland travelled away by air, Yvonne would drive to SickKids. This would be helpful for Yvonne; however, at times, it was challenging.

On several occasions, driving back home from SickKids, "I would be exhausted and tired, which led me to be extremely sleepy," Yvonne would later recall. "I would make a right turn and pull over into the parking lot of a plaza, stop the vehicle, turn the engine off, and put down my head on the steering wheel and take a short nap. Sometimes, I would wash my face with one of the water bottles that we normally keep in the minivan. I don't want to admit it, but I deeply believe that, sometimes, while driving from SickKids, I must have nodded off".

When Cleveland was not traveling by air, he would be driving to client sites, sometimes one hundred kilometers away from home. At those times, Yvonne would take public transit (trains and busses) to get Samantha to her appointments. And throughout these SickKids visits Pauline would babysit the other siblings – getting one on and off the school bus and staying at home with the other.

***** Sick Kids Visits July 2003 to November 2003 *****

JULY 2003

SUN	MON	TUES	WED	THURS	FRI	SAT
29	30	1	2	3 • Sick Kids trip • Blood works done • Platelet transfusion	4	5
6	7 • Sick Kids trip • Blood works done • Platelet transfusion	8	9	10	11	12
13	14 • Sick Kids trip • Blood works done • Platelet transfusion	15	16	17	18	19
20	21 • Sick Kids trip • Blood works done • Platelet transfusion	22	23 • Sick Kids trip • Blood works done • Platelet transfusion	24	25	26
27	28	29	30 • Sick Kids trip • Blood works done • Platelet transfusion	31		

We were happy to observe each sign of hope, and the much lower number of visits in August was the reason for joyous celebrations. We would take every sign of good news as major indications of hope.

AUGUST 2003

SUN	MON	TUES	WED	THURS	FRI	SAT
27	28	29	30	31	1	2
3	4	5	6	7	8	9
10	11 • Sick Kids trip • Blood works done • Platelet transfusion	12	13	14	15	16
17	18	19	20	21	22	23
24	25 • Sick Kids trip • Blood works done • Platelet transfusion	26	27	28	29	30

We had two visits in September 2003, on the 8th and 29th. We were delighted because, on both dates, Samantha's platelet counts were 127 and 178, respectively. Nothing was adequately big enough to contain the family's enormous joys. Below are copies of those CBC results.

```
                 Department of Paediatric Laboratory Medicine
          Phone: Core Laboratory 8800   Microbiology 6000   Blood Bank 6208

Patient:        STANBERRY,SAMANTHA YVONNE                DOB:    2001-03-22
HSC#:           2100777                                  Sex:    F
Location:       Haematology Service Clinic               Reg #:  A3081161
Responsible MD: Dror,Yigal
          Autosend Report (NOT a Chart Report) printed 2003-09-08 at 0937h

  M46687   COLL: 2003/09/08 09:23 REC: 2003/09/08 09:32 PHYS: Dror,Yigal


    CBC                                                              STAT
      WBC              L 2.7   4.3      (5.0-12.0)      X 10^9/L
      RBC              L 3.05           (4.00-5.00)     X 10^12/L
      HGB              L 95             (110-140)       g/L
      HCT              L 0.276          (0.350-0.420)
      MCV              90.3             (80.0-94.0)     fL
      MCH              31.0             (24.0-31.0)     pg
      MCHC             343              (320-360)       g/L
      PLT              L 127            (150-400)       X 10^9/L
      MPV              9.8              (4.0-14.0)      fL


                 Department of Paediatric Laboratory Medicine
          Phone: Core Laboratory 8800   Microbiology 6000   Blood Bank 6208

Patient:        STANBERRY,SAMANTHA YVONNE                DOB:    2001-03-22
HSC#:           2100777                                  Sex:    F
Location:       Haematology Service Clinic               Reg #:  A3095976
Responsible MD: Dror,Yigal
          Autosend Report (NOT a Chart Report) printed 2003-09-29 at 1003h

  M52227   COLL: 2003/09/29 09:30 REC: 2003/09/29 09:47 PHYS: Dror,Yigal


    CBC                                                              STAT
      WBC              L 2.7            (5.0-12.0)      X 10^9/L
      RBC              L 3.63           (4.00-5.00)     X 10^12/L
      HGB              115              (110-140)       g/L
      HCT              L 0.325          (0.350-0.420)
      MCV              89.5             (80.0-94.0)     fL
      MCH              H 31.6           (24.0-31.0)     pg
      MCHC             353              (320-360)       g/L
      PLT              178              (150-400)       X 10^9/L
      MPV              10.0             (4.0-14.0)      fL
```

The visits on October 20th and 27th had similar outcomes to September. Platelet counts were 127 and 137. November 10th and 17th were following the same trend of upwards and to the right. Platelet counts were 152 and 158, respectively. Up to this point, the platelet counts were slowly moving in a generally upward direction as the weeks and months went by. The results bounced back from the drop in October to the expected range by mid-November. We were really excited about this latest platelet count trajectory, as depicted below.

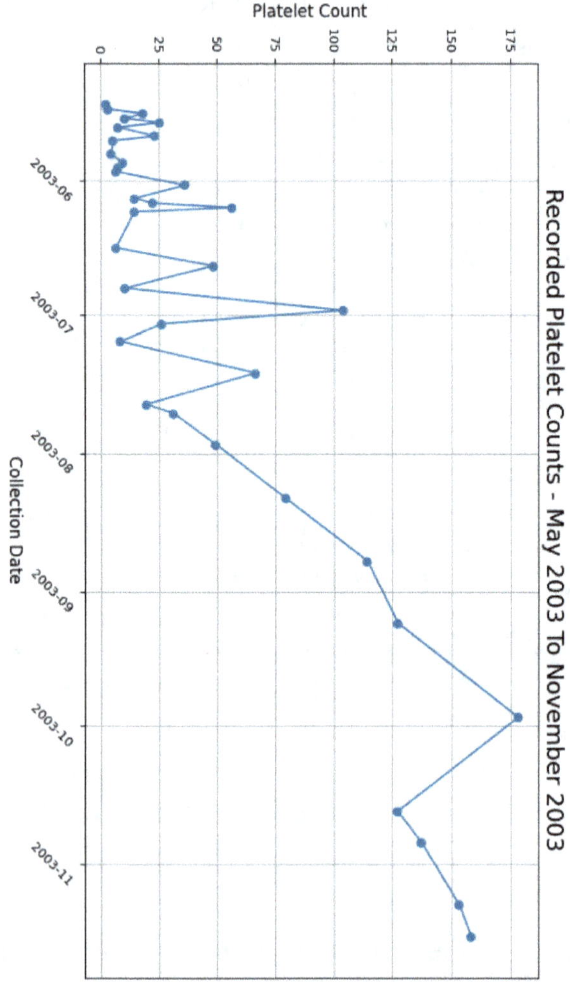

We started the month of December 2003 with high confidence and hope. On the December 1st visit, the results from the CBC showed platelet counts of 139, below the range of 150-400. However, for us, this was a highly satisfying and fulfilling result -

especially when compared to the counts of 2, 3, 6, 14, or even 48 in previous months.

Once the treatment with the cocktail of drugs started, there were conditions that we needed to be aware of. Samantha should not consume foods rich in potassium. This included bananas and other food. We believe that the reason was that food high in potassium would somehow interfere with the medications that she was on. Based on this guideline, Cranberry juice was the only satisfactory drink that we would have her consume. And, even then, it was only a particular brand and blend of cranberry juice with the lowest amount of potassium that would be suitable for her. This meant that we would meticulously look at food labels to observe if the nutritional information had any mention of potassium.

Also, we were advised that due to her lowered immune system because of the treatment, we should limit her exposure to germs or any organism that might make her become sick. We chose to not let her play outside and limit her contact with others outside of the home.

***** Get Ready For Christmas *****

Despite our best efforts, something caught up with Samantha. We didn't know what the culprit was, but at about 7:00 PM on December 22, 2003, Samantha came down with a bout of vomiting. Following the guidance to get to SickKids emergency if she experiences any symptoms, we arrived at SickKids emergency within an hour. As usual, it was another long night of CBC, but this time, she was treated for the vomiting, given platelets, and sent home at about 10:20 PM with instructions to continue her medications as prescribed. Below is the discharge form from that night.

-02   EMERX-6743
(QEMRE3)

THE HOSPITAL FOR SICK CHILDREN

STANBERRY, SAMANTHA YV
E3029293
2100777
2001-03-22
2003-12-22 21:04

EMERGENCY VISIT DISCHARGE INFORMATION SHEET

Child's regular doctor: DUIC, ANDREW D.

Discharge diagnosis: _______________________________

Your child has been assessed in the Emergency Department at The Hospital for Sick Children. This is an emergency assessment and diagnosis only. As it is often difficult to recognize and treat all aspects of any condition at a single visit, it is important that you follow the instructions listed below.

Instruction handouts given:
❏ Vomiting and Diarrhea   ❏ Febrile Seizure   ❏ Wound Care   ❏ Other:
❏ Asthma / Wheezing   ❏ Fever   ❏ Cast Care
❏ Head injury   ❏ Croup   ❏ Sedation

Medications:
• _______________________________
• _______________________________
• _______________________________

Other instructions:
____
____
____
____
____

❏ Follow up with your child's family doctor or paediatrician in ______ days, or sooner if necessary.
❏ A referral will be made to the _______________________ clinic.
❏ Lab results pending: _______________________
  ❏ We will call (positive results only)
  ❏ Check results with family doctor

If your child's condition is not improving or is worsening, you should contact your child's regular doctor. If you cannot reach your doctor, you may bring your child back to the Emergency Department, or you can obtain free medical telephone advice from Telehealth Ontario at 1-866-797-0000.

Your signature below indicates that you understand the information on this sheet.

_______________________   _______________________
Instructions given by   Parent, guardian, or patient's signature

Date: ____________   Time: ____________

White copy on chart   Yellow copy to patient

As we prepared to observe the usual Christmas and other holiday celebrations to close out the year, we were rather hopeful that things would continue to move in the right direction. Because of the vomiting on the 22nd, we chose to celebrate the holidays alone at home.

In the next few days, from December 23rd to 25th, we spent time preparing a special meal that has become our own family Christmas tradition. For appetizers, lobster bisque and freshly baked dinner rolls. The main course includes smoked ham and braised lamb shanks. This was paired with mushrooms stuffed with spinach and parmesan cheese, roasted potatoes, and homemade sorrel drink.

Dessert was Yvonne's Jamaican fruit cake (also known as rum cake), using prunes, dates, currants, and raisins that have been soaking in Jamaican white rum for the past year. Indeed, we've always had a batch soaking in a jar – even up to this day!

Except for Samantha, we all enjoyed the appetizer, main course, and dessert. We took it upon ourselves not to share the pleasure of eating the fruit cake with her because even though we believed 99% of the alcohol was lost during the baking process, we just didn't want to take any chances with her. We had hoped that sometime in the future, she could have all the fruit cake that she wanted to have.

New Year's Eve came around with the usual celebrations. We stayed home and watched the celebrations on television as various places around the world moved away from 2003 and welcomed January 1, 2004, with hopes and dreams. We watched as many said goodbye to the old year and imagined better times in the new year. Lovers kissed, some got engaged, others frolicked as best as they could.

But everyone we saw on television seemed to have bright hopes for 2004. Some wore oversized 2004 glasses while they partied in New York and other cities. The emotion on some faces suggested that they were brushing off the trials of the past year and replacing them with expected triumphs of the coming new year as they ushered in 2004.

Would our family also move from the trials of 2003 and revel in future triumphs of 2004? Looking back at 2003, we could see some good signs. We started 2003 with a single-income mock budget and by May 2003, it had become the real-life budget. We were still making ends meet. Samantha's platelets were generally moving upwards and to the right, in the region of 140 – 400, the counts that are considered normal. We would return to the folder holding the records to give ourselves hope. Below is the chart of the recorded platelet counts from the day of diagnosis, May 15th, 2003, to our final CBC record of 2003 (December 15th, 2003).

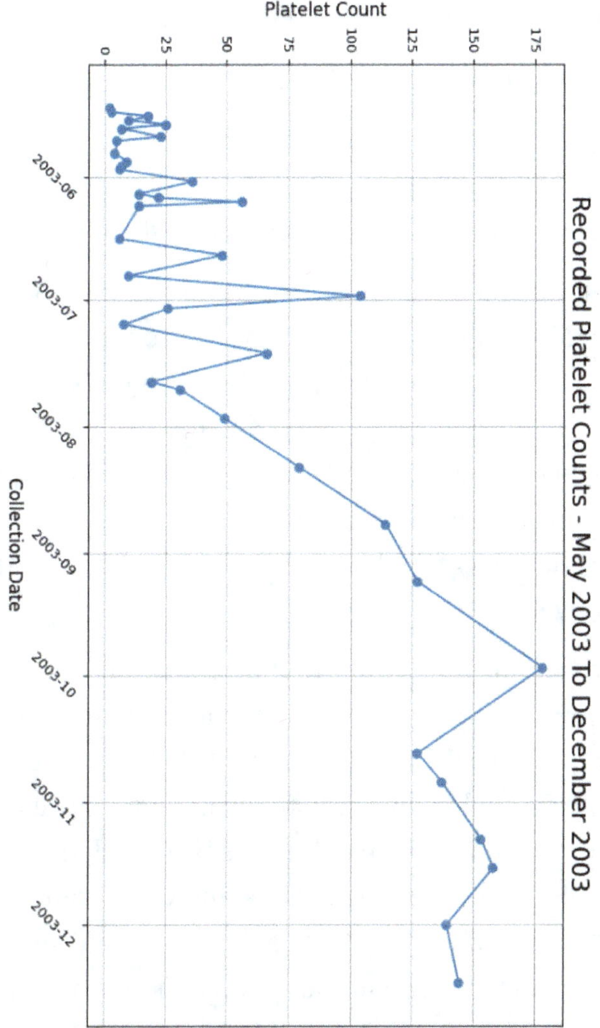

Indeed 2004 started better than the middle of 2003. Based on the records given to us by SickKids, we have observed the following.

May 15, 2003, to December 31, 2003

- Samantha was at SickKids doing CBC investigations an average of every 6 days.

- Most visits included platelet transfusion

May 3, 2004, to December 31, 2004

- Samantha was at SickKids doing CBC investigations an average of every 24 days.
- Fewer visits included platelet transfusion

This meant that we made less frequent visits to SickKids. This was a good indicator. For the family, improvements happened. By June 2004, Cleveland changed his job, and his income doubled. By now we outlived and out-performed the mock-budget. He would travel locally more often, and this meant that if he were away driving to clients, then Yvonne would need another vehicle to get to SickKids within an hour if Samantha showed any symptoms.

The increased income meant that he could buy another car. Yvonne now had the minivan to shuttle Samantha to SickKids at a moment's notice. Being home meant that the children enjoyed warm oven home-baked bread to go along with sausage because luckily (or blessed) for them, Yvonne loved baking and made bread almost twice per week. Cleveland would only come home in the evenings to hear the tales of how the children had sumptuous lunches and snacks of warm home-baked bread and sausages.

2004 was not without its challenges, however. Before June 2004, prior to the second car being bought, Yvonne would struggle at times on the busses and subway trains to get to SickKids during times when Cleveland was away on work-related road trips.

***** The Party That Wasn't To Be *****

Other challenges followed us to December 2004. On the morning of Saturday December 11, 2004, we noticed pimples on the back and head of Samantha. These were different from the spots that we saw in May 2003, so we just thought this was not related to Aplastic Anemia.

We decided that Cleveland would take Samantha to her pediatrician, Dr. Duic. We thought that this would be routine because, on the 29th of November 2004, her platelet counts were 188, well within the range of 140 to 400. We might have been overconfident, thinking that this should be a quick test to validate that she is still doing okay. Well, if anything can go wrong, sometimes they will. And today, things will go wrong.

Dr. Duic immediately sent her to SickKids Emergency. So, Cleveland and Samantha made the trip to SickKids Emergency. She was assessed and eventually admitted. The diagnosis was Chicken Pox. With her compromised immune system, we were thankful that the clinicians were not taking any risks. She was given Tylenol due to a fever of 39°C. The antiviral drug Acyclovir was given intravenously. The next day, December 12th, Hydroxyzine was started to stop the itching. The copy below is handwritten notes taken from the 11th and 12th.

December 11, 2004

Pimples Noticed in head & back
Taken to Dr. Dulic – Dr. Dulic referred her
Sick Kids Emerg.
⇒ Chicken Pox Diagnosed initially
⇒ Had fever of 39.0 given Tylenol
⇒ Antiviral Acyclovir given intravenously
350 mg in 58 ml = concentration (every 8hrs

⇒ Vomited before Acyclovir was given

⇒ Dr. Williams (dermatologist) – it may be chicken pox
or herpes

– December 12, 2004
– Dr. .... ~~Hydroxyzine~~ Hydroxyzine 10 MG every 8
to stop itching.
– Fever was 39.5 @ 7:55pm. – receive Tylenol

It was during the hospitalization that it was noticed with one of the CBCs that there were some problems with renal function. As we would later learn, Samantha's kidney function was minimal. Below is a summary of this, yet another hospitalization discharge form.

```
7BX  -5269           THE HOSPITAL FOR SICK CHILDREN
2004-12-16  11:15           (QNOLKP-014-043- JMDH)              PAGE 001
                         DISCHARGE ORDER/SUMMARY

STANBERRY, SAMANTHA                         HSC#: 2100777
DOB: 2001-03-22                             WEIGHT(KG): 16.8
ADMIT DATE: 2004-12-11                      UNIT: 7B
SERVICE: PAEDIATRIC MED. PHONE: 416-813-6921   ADMIT#: I4010210
HSC RESPONSIBLE PHYSICIAN: BERNSTEIN, STACEY MD
HSC CONTACT: NOT AVAIL.                      PHONE: NOT AVAIL.
_______________________________________________________________________

DISCHARGE TODAY (2004-12-16).
MD TO SEE PATIENT PRIOR TO DISCHARGE, (JMDH)


ALLERGIES:
   MED ALLERGIES
      2003-05-16   NO MEDICATION ALLERGIES KNOWN
   DIET ALLERGIES
      2003-05-16   NO FOOD ALLERGIES KNOWN
_______________________________________________________________________

   DISCHARGE CONTINGENT UPON:
   DISCHARGE CONTINGENT UPON: TEMPERATURE NORMAL

   MOST RESPONSIBLE DIAGNOSIS:
   VARICELLA ZOSTER (CHICKENPOX)

   OTHER DIAGNOSIS:
   APLASTIC ANEMIA
   RENAL IMPAIRMENT

   DISCHARGE MEDICATIONS:
   CYCLOSPORINE NEORAL 75 MG BY MOUTH 2TIMES DAILY QUANTITY:ONE MONTH
   SUPPLY REPEATS:THREE
   ACYCLOVIR PO 340 MG BY MOUTH 4TIMES DAILY FOR 4 DAYS QUANTITY:FOUR
   DAY SUPPLY

   DIET:
   USUAL DIET

   HOSPITAL COURSE/INVESTIGATION RESULTS:
       ADM WITH NEW ONSET OF CUTANEOUS VESICLES. WAS NOTED TO HAVE
   DECREASED RENAL FUNCTION ON THE INITIAL LAB. THOUGHT TO BE
   SECONDARY TO CYCLOSPORIN. CYCLOSPORIN HELD AND ACYCLOVIR IV
   STARTED. DOSES ADJUSTED FOR RENAL FUNC. PT WELL KNOWN TO HEME
   SRVC-DR DROR. CYCLOSPORIN RESUMED DUE TO THE PT BEING KNOWN TO
   RELAPSE EASILY WHEN TAKEN OFF CYCLO.
       DURING HER STAY, SAMANTHA BECAME FEBRILE. BLOOD CULTURES TAKEN
   WHICH ARE (-) TO DATE. LESIONS DID NOT SHOW ANY SIGNS OF SECONDARY
   BAC INFEC. FEVER WAS THOUGHT TO BE SECONDARY TO VIRAL INFECTION.
   LESIONS STARTED TO CRUST AN NO NEW LESIONS APPEARED. INITIALLY HAD

                            CONTINUED

=======================================================================
STANBERRY, SAMANTHA YVONNE  2100777              DISCHARGE ORDER/SUMM
```

We were told that there could be multiple implications, and so it needed to be dealt with. This resulted in Samantha seeing a nephrologist (kidney function doctor) for the next ten years. Fortunately, Dr. Pearl was located on the ground floor of the SickKids hospital, so going to appointments to see her was in a familiar place. One implication is that the development of puberty could be severely impacted. It was rather interesting to observe the delight and excitement of her father when Samantha had her first period. "Never could I have known that a man would be so excited that his daughter is having her first period," Yvonne would later quip.

Throughout the day of the chicken pox ordeal on December 11th, Cleveland was calling home to get Yvonne. However, she didn't pick up after several calls. He only reached her when he arrived at SickKids, and Samantha was hospitalized by then. Yvonne drove to the hospital, and Cleveland returned home to relieve Pauline, who was babysitting the other two children. Yvonne and Samantha would remain in the hospital for almost a week before they were discharged on December 16th, 2004.

On Cleveland's next visit to Samantha the next day (Sunday), Yvonne told him how she was somewhat relieved that he was making what we thought was a quick trip to Dr. Duic because she had planned a surprise for him.

She explained that she had planned a surprise birthday party for him, and she was, at times, out busy with her secret plans with family and some friends. She picked up the voicemails I had left on her return and then quickly called all the guests that she had invited to tell them that she had to cancel the party because the trip to SickKids turned out to be more than we had hoped. Cleveland appreciated the gesture. He still has the gift from Yvonne's friend Pamella, a tie, to this day.

He would later that week consume more than half of the Jamaican fruit cake that Yvonne baked for the party. But poor Samantha couldn't have any because the prunes, dates, and currants that are primary ingredients were soaked in Jamaican overproof white rum for more than six months (we always have these soaking in the fridge, even up to this day!).

December 2004 indeed ended on a better note. Yvonne could get to the hospital faster and more comfortably. She would have less stress with the busses and trains of the public transportation system. Above all, it appears that the treatment was working because, in 2004, Samantha's platelet counts continued where they were at the end of 2003 and continued to remain close to or within the range of 140 to 400 for the last month of 2004.

We love the colored plot that compares the platelet counts in 2003 with those in 2004, as shown below. It shows that her platelet counts remained mostly in the band between 100 and 250 for the duration of our record-keeping up to the end of 2004.

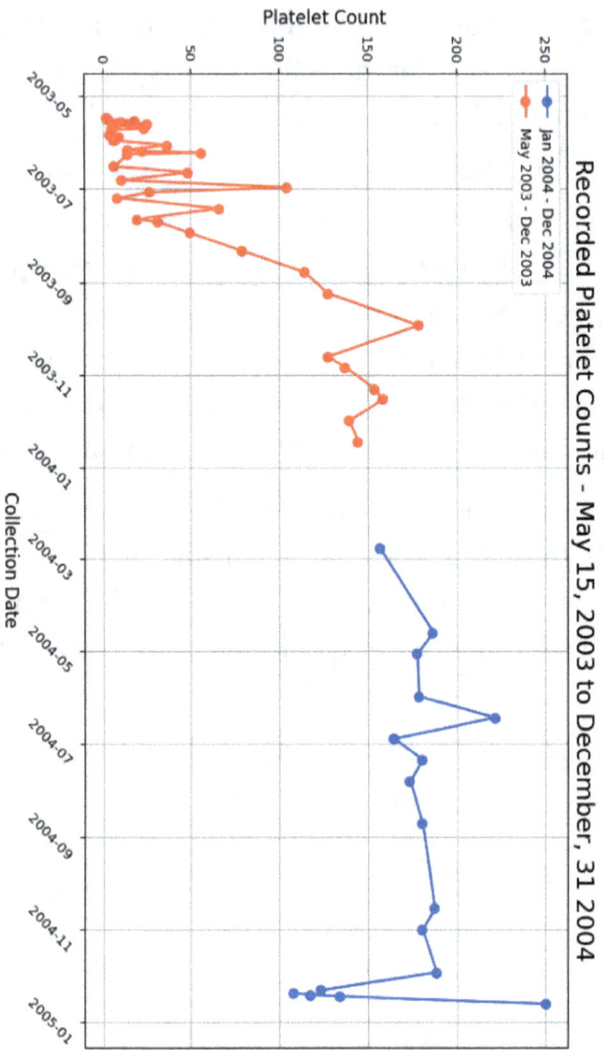

Samantha would continue to be treated with cyclosporin for the next six years. Her appointment schedule for CBC was now about every three months. During this time, the cyclosporin dosage was tapered each month and lowered to a very small dosage - 0.05 ml - during the final month. During the final three months, a long, slender syringe was used to measure each dosage. Her last dosage was in November 2009.

She continued to have scheduled CBC tests every two to three months after the end of the cyclosporin treatment. This continued until October 2010. The frequency of scheduled CBC testing was moved out to every six months starting in April 2011, and lasting up to October 2016.

The steady improvement in her platelet counts gave us hope. While most people offered genuine support, we had to shield ourselves from those whose words brought pain rather than comfort. We remember two women who came to pray for our daughter – their initial kindness turned bitter when they suggested our sins had caused her illness. Whatever 'sin' is, we are yet to find it recorded in the medical journals that it causes Aplastic Anemia. Others superstitiously claimed that with twins, one child was destined to die.

But these dark moments were far outweighed by the community that rallied around us. Friends, family, and even people unknown to us became beacons of strength, doing everything in their power to lift our spirits during these challenging times.

After October 3, 2016, scheduled CBC tests were conducted yearly. The Aplastic Anemia would continue to be managed by SickKids up to March 2019, because SickKids treats patients up to age eighteen. After this age, patients are referred to the Toronto cancer centers at Princess Margaret Hospital or Sunnybrook Hospital. Sunnybrook was selected by us as the center to continue the management of the disease.

During the final scheduled appointment at SickKids in March 2019, we sought out each of the staff and thanked them for their many years of support. Samantha expressed her gratitude to Dr. Dror for his fifteen years of effective and dedicated care, plus his exceptional treatment management of her rare disease. She presented him with a framed portrait with the words Severe Acute Aplastic Anemia. Samantha took about a week to develop the concept and complete the portrait. A copy of the portrait is below.

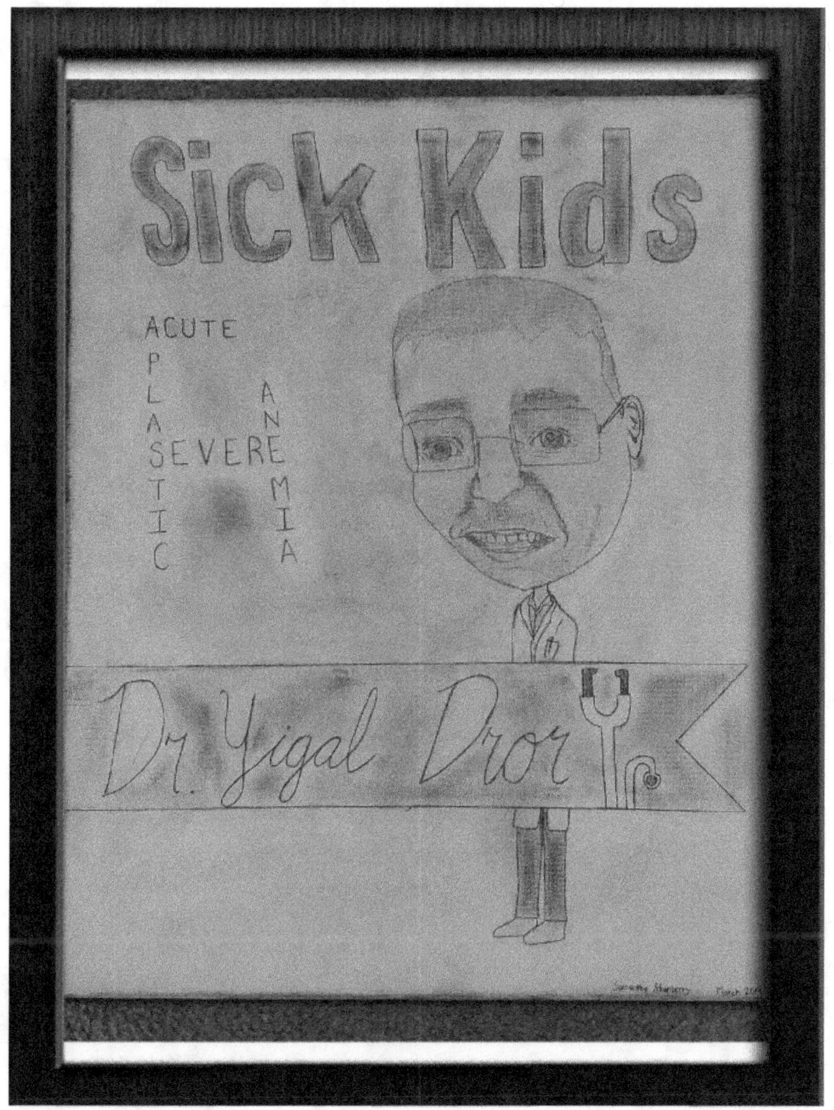

Portrait of Samantha's primary care physician, presented to him in March 2019

Her last platelet count on June 21, 2024, was 145. While at the lower level, we are grateful that it is within the expected range. Below is a graphical overview of the important platelet counts, reproduced from some of the twenty-one years of actual hospital records - from May 15, 2003, to June 21, 2024.

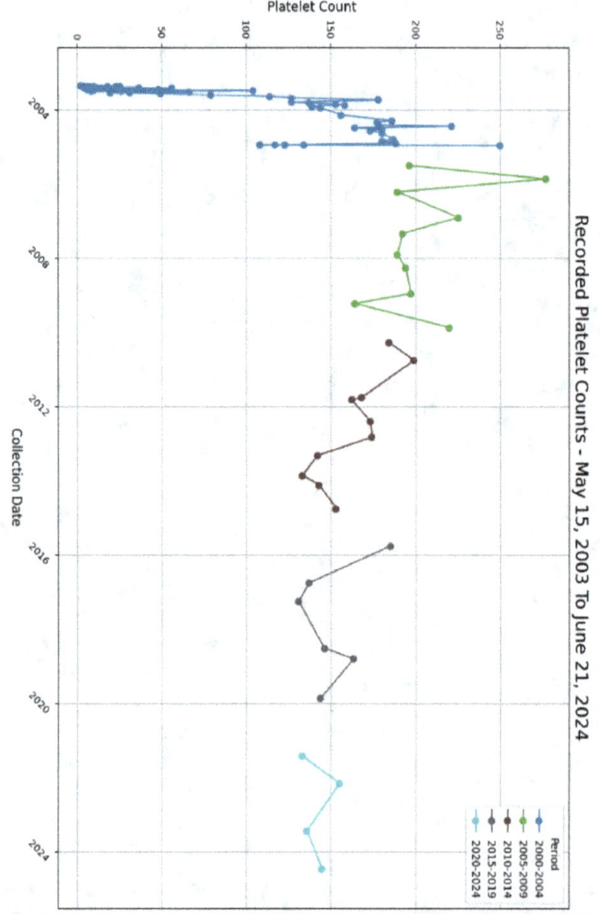

Yvonne seemed to have beaten the clock that was ticking on May 15th, 2003, as she vowed to do.

5

The Big Lie (The School Years)

In 2002, we sold and moved from the condominium that we lived in since 1998. We bought and moved into a newly built three-bedroom semi-detached house. We were excited to see it being built from the ground up. On weekends, we would visit the site to see progress. We observed its evolution from the excavation of the basement to the building of its foundation.

We watched the gradual construction of the inner and outer walls to the new shingles on the roof. We upgraded the main floor parquet hardwood, we selected the tiles for the kitchen, and for the upper floor, we selected thicker and upgraded carpet under pads, chose the carpet color, and for the main, floor we selected upgraded appliances. We upgraded the bathroom to a Mirolin-branded tub with six jets. We even customized the inside by working with the builder to create a narrow wall that separated the foyer from the living room – this provided more privacy when viewed from the outside. We were emotionally invested in the new house.

The twin girls were glad to continue to be together, sharing one of the rooms, while our son had his own room. Yvonne graciously shared her room with Cleveland. We were contented. However, we would soon realize that all moments of contentment may just be fleeting times of temporary fulfillment. We would learn to enjoy those moments while they lasted.

In 2004, when our first child was in elementary school, he began bringing home homework assignments. He would do his homework at the dinner table. However, if the television was playing in the adjoining family room, or there was a visitor having a conversation in the kitchen or living room, or Cleveland was playing the piano, the sounds would be too loud for the child to concentrate on doing his homework. And we wanted other members of the family to also carry on with their lives.

Driven by this observation, we decided that we would dedicate a room in the house for schoolwork. The basement was not a choice because Cleveland worked from home two to three days per week, and that's where his office was located. For that reason, we decided that we needed a house with four bedrooms. We would repurpose one of the bedrooms as a library, the twin girls would continue to share a room, our son would have his own room, and fortunately for Cleveland, he could continue to share a room with Yvonne. The idea was that Cleveland would create an office space in the basement.

In July 2005, we sold and moved out of the semi-customized three-bedroom house into a four-bedroom property that provided us with our desires. It gave us all that we wished for. There was a room in the completed, carpeted basement with ample bookshelves suitable for Cleveland's office. The bedroom most suitable for the library was above the dining room – perhaps the quietest place during the evenings.

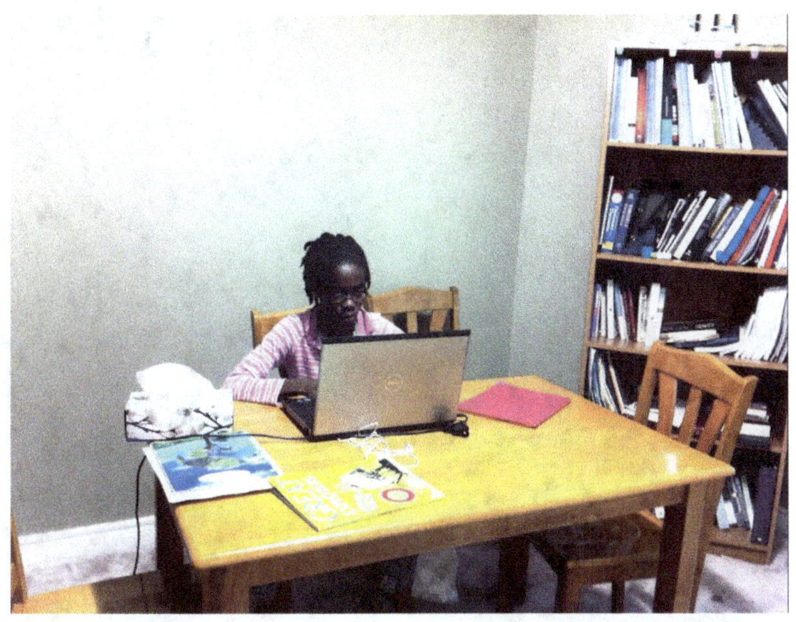

Picture of Antoinette working in the library (in September 2012)

For the library upstairs, shown as bedroom 2 in the actual builder schematic below, we bought a small four-seater wooden dining table and placed it in the center of the room. We bought three wooden bookcases that matched the natural color of the table. Later, within two years, these bookcases would be stacked with children's books. The overflow books rested on top of the shelves and in bins on the floor. There were books, books everywhere - mathematics, English, geography, French, science, and several Robert Munsch books. Cleveland would end up complaining that he can't walk in the library because he's constantly tripping over books. But that was a small inconvenience because, at least, everything we planned for was achieved. Or were they?

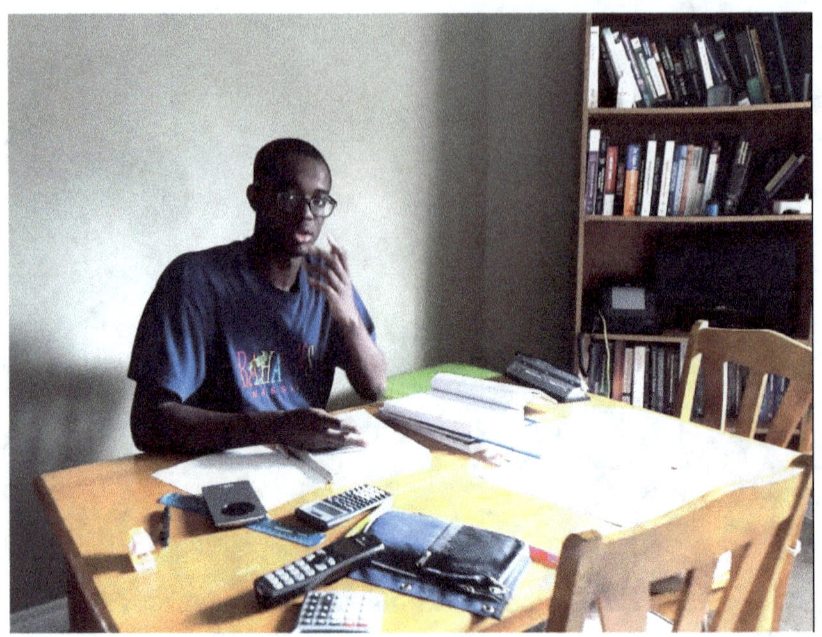

Picture of Clive-Anthony studying in the library (in September 2015)

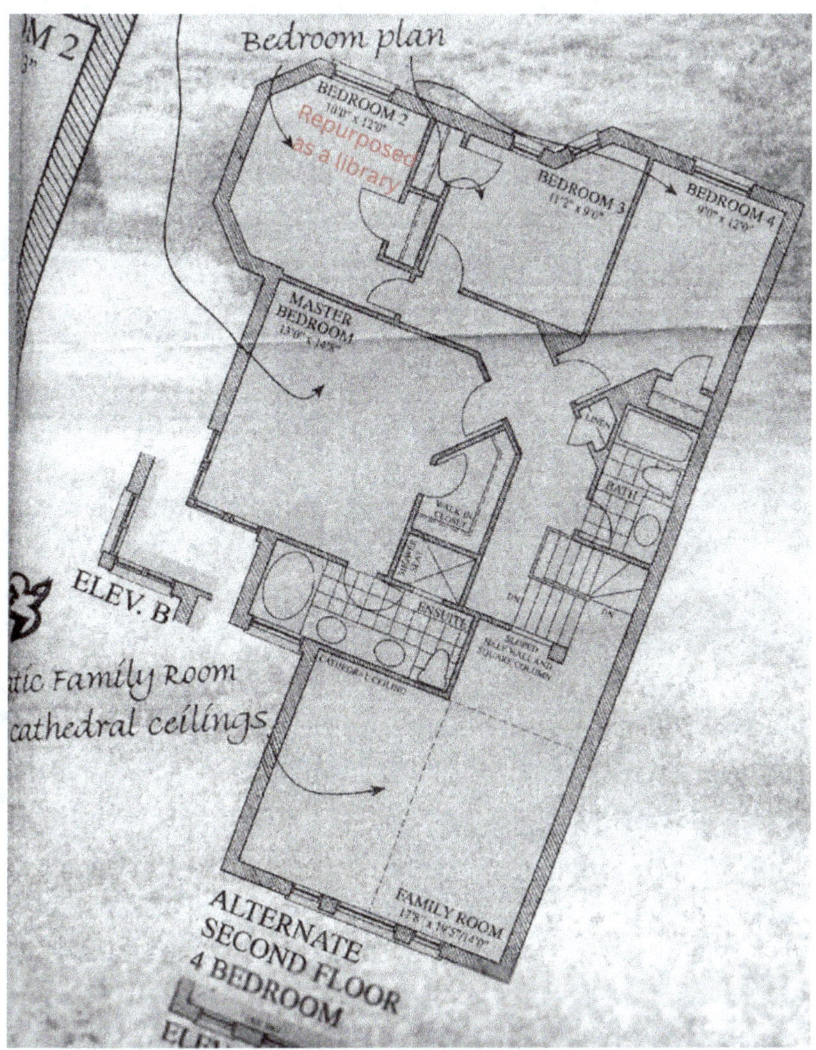

Actual builder's blueprint of a house in which we repurposed bedroom 2 as a library

Two years after moving to the new house, during the summer of 2007, on July 31st, all five of us went to Samantha's scheduled appointment at SickKids. This was another routine visit that we treated as a family outing because the other two children were on their summer break from school. Samantha's two siblings,

Antoinette and Clive-Anthony were more excited about the play area in the clinic than any other thing going on around them. We were excited for other reasons. The CBC results from that visit showed that Samantha's platelet counts were 204. This was good news indeed.

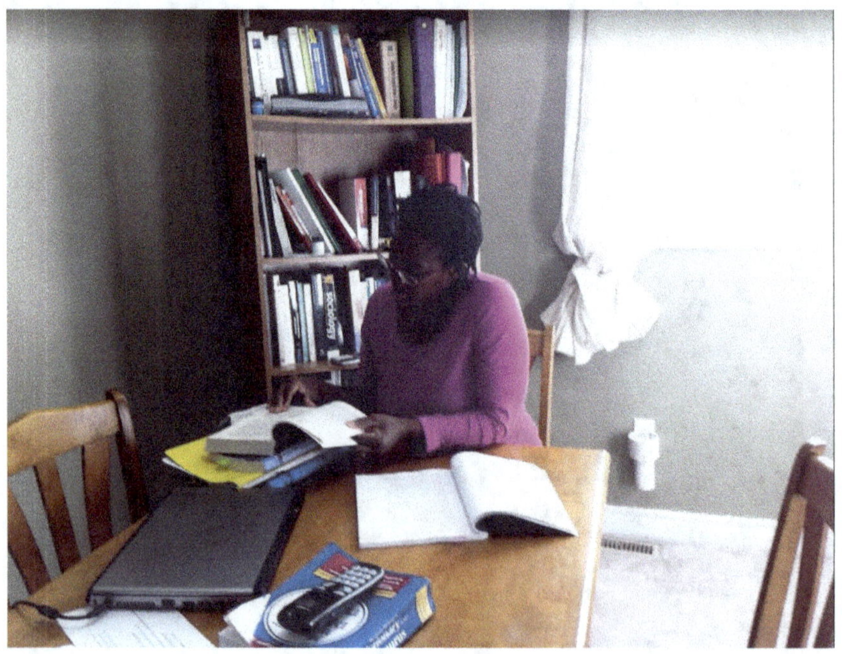

Picture of Yvonne studying in the library (9:14 AM, Tuesday, October 22, 2013)

We packed into the minivan and left the hospital for home. Traveling south on Bay Street, we soon arrived under the bridge several meters south of Front Street West. At that moment, Clive-Anthony shouted out the question, "Daddy, why is that man sleeping under the bridge?". Cleveland quickly looked to his right to see someone lying down under the bridge on what appeared to be cardboard.

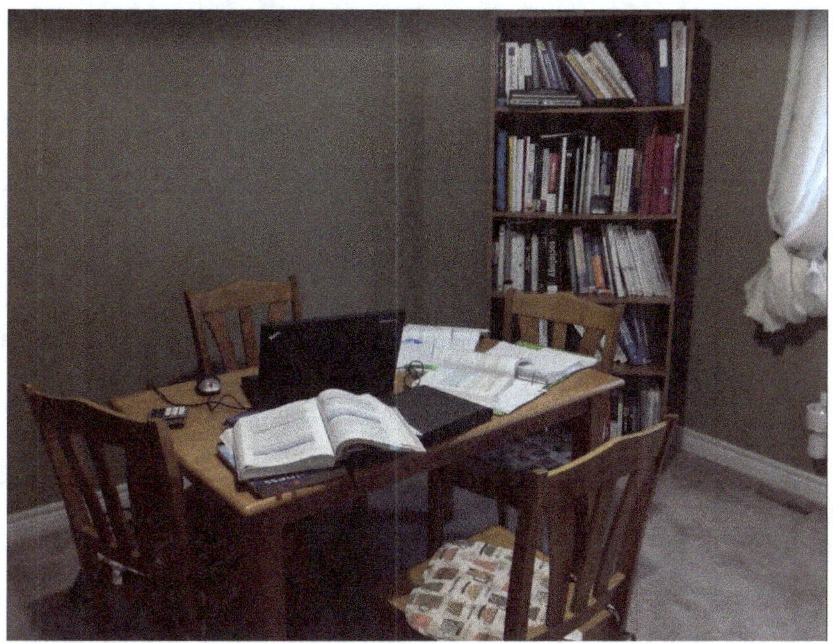

Samantha was missing in this picture of the library in December 2013 – likely, she was at SickKids Hospital!

We all waited with bated breath for his answer. By this time, we must have approached the ramp to the Gardiner Expressway, and we didn't get an answer. Clearly, two to four minutes must have passed since the question was asked. Why was he taking so long to respond? Later that evening Cleveland would confess that he didn't want to tell his son that he didn't know the truthful answer to the question.

And then the response came. "He didn't do his homework," Cleveland said with confidence. He said it with the kind of dogma that one would hear spewing from the mouth of politicians to their constituents when they are running to get elected. To everyone in the vehicle, this seemed to be a fact not to be questioned, as if it were indisputable.

"So, if you don't do your homework, you'll end up sleeping under a bridge?" the young, impressionable Clive-Anthony asked, in a child-like tone characterized by pure innocence. Here comes the supporting lie. "Yes", Cleveland responded.

Clive-Anthony wept all the way home.

We came to later understand that the impact of this "big lie" transformed Clive-Anthony's approach to life, and with this approach, he influenced the minds and attitudes of his sisters.

Later in the autumn of that year, 2007, during the new school term, Cleveland happened to be passing by the girls' room when he heard Clive-Anthony whispering, "Girls, you better do your homework so that you don't sleep under a bridge." Cleveland quickly went downstairs and relayed to Yvonne what he just heard. Both Cleveland and Yvonne were surprised that Clive-Anthony remembered the lie. Being a young child, they didn't know that the lie had such an impact on him that he would be telling his sisters to steer clear of doing something that could lead to sleeping under a bridge.

Early the next year, Samantha came downstairs to the kitchen crying and said, "Mommy, Antoinette doesn't want to do her homework, and I don't want her to live under a bridge." Yvonne turned off the stove and went upstairs to the library with Samantha in tow, following close behind me. Antoinette was walking around in the library with no care in the world. Yvonne said to Antoinette, "Antoinette, look at your sister; she's in tears. She just told me that you don't want to do your homework, and she is crying because she doesn't want you to live under a bridge".

Yvonne continued, "Antoinette, do you have homework?". "Yes, Mommy," she responded. Yvonne said, "Well, Antoinette, it's time to do your homework. And make sure you finish your homework before supper. Always do your homework when you get home from school".

That was the last time that Yvonne had a conversation with the children about homework for the remainder of their elementary, high school, or even university years.

The lesson we learned was that the big lie transcended the boundary of the minivan. It was embedded into the consciousness of Clive-Anthony. He pushed it into Samantha's awareness, and Samantha was so taken up with the connection between not doing homework and sleeping under a bridge that she wept when faced with the reality that her sister was not doing her homework.

The attitude towards engaging in school was hopefully embedded deep within our children at this time. Next, let's hear from them about their school years.

***** Clive-Anthony's Schooling *****

My educational journey was profoundly shaped by what my family now calls "the big lie" - my father's impromptu explanation about a homeless person sleeping under a bridge. That single moment in the summer of 2007, when I was still in elementary school, became the cornerstone of my academic motivation. The simple yet impactful statement, "He didn't do his homework," created a ripple effect that influenced not just my approach to education but also my sisters' attitudes toward their studies.

I remember vividly how that car ride home from SickKids Hospital changed everything. After seeing that man under the bridge and hearing my father's explanation, I wept the entire way home. The connection between education and life outcomes became crystal clear in my young mind - perhaps too clear. I took it upon myself to become not just a dedicated student but also a guardian of sorts for my sisters' academic success. I would whisper warnings to them about the importance of doing homework, sharing the cautionary tale that had so deeply affected me.

My formal education began at age four at Huntington Ridge Public School in Mississauga, Canada, where I attended Junior Kindergarten. The following year, I moved to Levy Creek Public School for Senior Kindergarten before continuing my elementary education at Vista Heights Public School.

Each summer, my mother would buy English and mathematics books for the upcoming grade that we would be moving into the upcoming September. We had to work through most chapters of those books at least one hour after breakfast each day during the months of July and August.

It was during these early years that our family's dedication to education led them to choose a four-bedroom house specifically to create a dedicated library room for our studies. This room, positioned above the dining room to ensure quiet, became our academic sanctuary.

Since my early days at Levy Creek Public School, I discovered that I loved mathematics. It was so logical, and at that time, I particularly liked problems that had anything to do with patterns. At Vista Heights, I discovered my love for athletics, participating in both basketball and track and field.

I continued to excel in mathematics at Vista Heights, scoring 100% on many of our tests. I remember how excited I was when, the same evening that I took home my third consecutive one hundred percent math test score, my dad took us to the store to pay about two hundred dollars for my first pair of Nike basketball shoes. This was to reward me for achieving math scores of 100% three times in a row. At the time, I didn't fully understand why my parents were more focused on rewarding me for academic success when some of my other friends were given twelve pairs of Nike basketball shoes to go with each month of the year – just for being offsprings. I now better understand their reasoning.

My friend Taylor also excelled in mathematics. Sometimes, our grade 6 teacher, Mr. McCaughey, would give us advanced work to complete while he taught the class. He would often say that he was sure that I would become an actuary. I was one hundred percent sure that he was wrong because my friend Taylor and I made a pact that we would study medicine when we reached university. Life, however, had different plans in store.

My journey continued at Green Glade Sr. Public School, where I continued to excel in mathematics and, surprisingly also, French. The Core French program meant many of our subjects were taught in French, and I thrived in this bilingual environment. My passion for basketball continued as I played on the school team, taking care of only taking out my Nike shoes on game days.

High school at St. Aloysius Gonzaga Secondary School marked a period of intense academic dedication. However, I lost my passion for French education but maintained my passion for mathematics. I completed 34 subjects during regular day school, including mathematics, physics, chemistry, biology, philosophy, and music.

My drive for academic excellence led me to attend summer school for three consecutive years, completing two English courses and one Civics course during the summer months. This accelerated pace allowed me to fulfill all requirements for my high school diploma by January 2015, several months ahead of the expected June graduation.

This freedom allowed me to accompany my dad to a university conference in Ottawa, at which he was presenting a paper. I took the liberty to ask one of the presenters a question about the p-value in his statistical analysis. During the lunch break, some professors in attendance were shocked that I was still in high school and could understand the materials being discussed and being able to pose the question about p-value.

Beyond academics, I immersed myself in various activities. As a member of the high school band playing the tuba, I had the incredible opportunity to tour Europe, visiting England, Scotland, and Ireland. I played intramural Canadian football for a year and maintained my involvement in intramural basketball and volleyball throughout high school, eventually becoming an assistant coach for the girls' basketball team.

A pivotal moment in my academic journey came when I read Michio Kaku's "Physics of the Future" from my father's collection. A book that he specifically forbids me to read. I now believe that he really intended for me to read the book but was playing mind games with me. The book's predictions about technology's role in medicine led me to reconsider my earlier plan to study medicine. Instead, I became fascinated with the idea of being involved in the technology that would inform physicians - data science.

In Fall 2014, before graduating high school, I applied to five universities - four in Canada for Biology, Biochemistry, and Mathematics programs, and one in the UK at the University of London for Mathematics and Economics. Thanks to my parents' support in paying the application fees, I was able to cast a wide net and was accepted into all five schools. Although my true passion was data science, it wasn't offered as a program at the time. I ultimately chose to study Mathematics and Economics through the University of London's distance learning program, beginning in October 2015.

While my parents funded my first year of university, I took responsibility for my education expenses thereafter. I worked various jobs to support my education journey and for my leisure activities: as a bank teller, a lifeguard, and a first aid trainer. In an amusing twist, one of my high school teachers ended up being a student in one of my first-aid classes. I even started my own first-aid training company, conducting sessions in my parents' basement. My costs were low because I didn't pay them for the use of the basement.

It was not only my income from the various part-time jobs that funded my university fees. Our parents instilled investing in us starting from our grade-school days, and through capital gains from those investments, I comfortably paid my way through my undergraduate studies.

These investment strategies proved so effective that within six months of my move to the US, I was a proud homeowner. I look forward to sharing the full story of my financial journey in a dedicated book, where I will delve into the specific techniques and strategies that made it possible.

Through this combination of work, investment, and study, I managed to complete my undergraduate degree without any student debt.

***** Antoinette's Schooling *****

My schooling began at Levy Creek Public School in Mississauga. Although my memories of this early period are somewhat hazy, I remember clearly that my sister Sam and I didn't share the same classroom. At lunchtime, I would make a hasty dash out the door to find her. I can also remember it marked the start of my lifelong love for art and drawing.

After we moved to another house in Mississauga, I continued my elementary education at Vista Heights Public School from senior kindergarten through to the fifth grade. During summer breaks, our mother instilled a strong work ethic in us. We diligently completed book reports and spent an hour each morning focused on math and English lessons from the curriculum of the upcoming school year. However, the remainder of the day was dedicated to carefree play, often involving climbing the large tree in our backyard and losing ourselves in books. I was also an active child, participating in cross-country and track at Vista Heights Public School.

In sixth grade, I transitioned to Divine Mercy Catholic Elementary School. This proved to be an excellent choice, as I thrived academically and athletically. I joined the cross-country, volleyball, and basketball teams, and we proudly brought home two school championships. I entered a competition to design the team logo for the 2013 to 2014 school year, and I won the competition. My creation is shown below for the team logo selected, and I still cherish the jersey bearing my creation to this day.

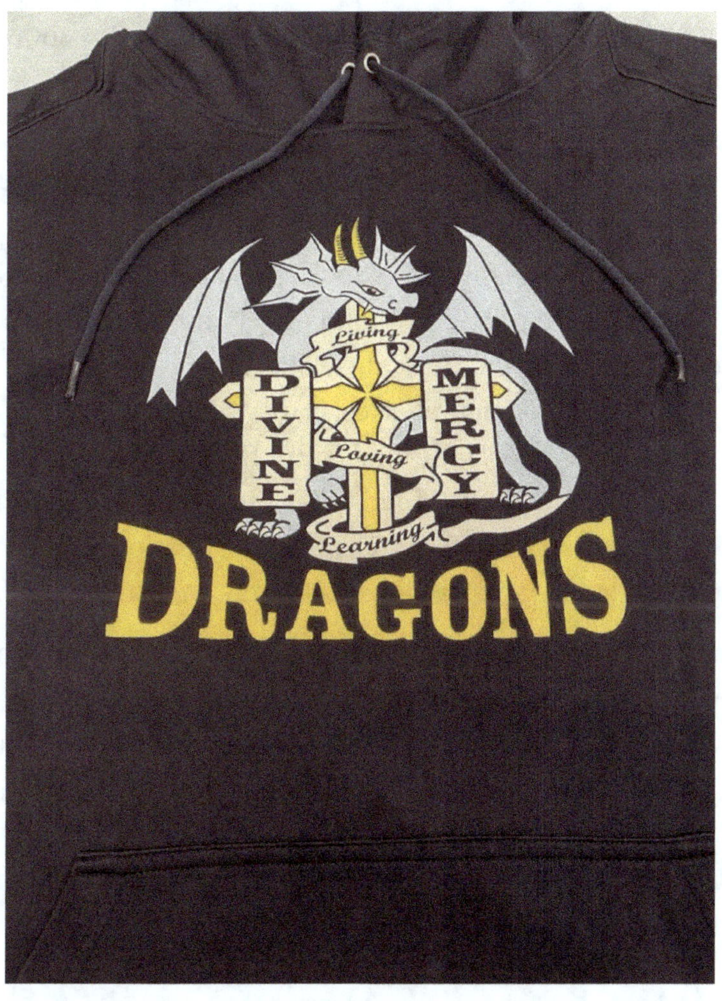

Antoinette middle-school artwork on Divine Mercy School jersey

My sister and I were dedicated athletes, and our mother's enthusiastic support from the stands was always a source of motivation.

At St. Aloysius Gonzaga Secondary School, I continued my involvement in sports, playing on the volleyball and basketball teams. However, my focus shifted to academics, particularly mathematics, physics, and computer science. Through diligent summer school attendance, I accelerated my studies and was accepted into the University of London in March 2019.

From 2006 and up to the end of high school, our family vacations were a highlight of the summers. However, we still had to take our math and English books with us. I enjoyed many trips to Canadian destinations such as Blue Mountain Ski Resort, Deerhurst Resort and Great Wolf Lodge. American destinations included the Cleveland Rock and Roll Hall of Fame, the winding Lombard Street in San Francisco, Napa Valley, Disney's Animal Kingdom Lodge in Orlando, and South Beach in Miami, Florida. European adventures included Paris and riding on the under-sea train from Paris to London. Caribbean destinations included a couple of trips to Jamaica and several more to Saint Martin.

Since high school, my dad would teach us about investments. He would often say that saving money is not good – a strange idea, we would think. It's better to invest money; he would often argue at the dinner table. With income from my lifeguard job and investment returns, I was able to significantly finance my university education. I look forward to sharing more about my investment journey in a future publication.

It seems that most of what we learned from our parents was at the dining table because, since my earliest memories, we almost always had dinners together.

Saturday breakfasts and Sunday dinners were especially the targeted occasions for refined home dining. On Saturdays, we'd gather for a formal breakfast, setting our dining room table with our most exquisite carafe, teapots, teacups, cutlery, and plateware. The meal was mostly Jamaican soul food that would include ackee and salt fish, kale, spinach, swiss chard, fried plantains, and boiled green bananas, served with hibiscus and other herbal teas. We would look forward to personalized fried dumplings shaped in the letters that start our first names, A, S, C, and Y.

Sunday dinners would be equally elegant, featuring a three-course meal, starting many times with salads, roasted butternut squash soup, or my mom's obsession - lobster bisque. On trips to Canada's east coast, my dad would often return with live lobsters in a box, and mom would boil and freeze them, making them last for as long as possible to make even more lobster bisque. I would be remiss not to mention the fluffy, mouthwatering homemade dinner rolls or cheddar biscuits that my mom would often make.

The main course would include rice and peas, roasted potatoes paired with broiled salmon, broiled T-bone steak, roasted chicken, braised lamb shanks, or our favorite ground beef casserole. It was a joy for my sister and me to help make the béchamel for the casserole by continuously stirring the milk while whisking in the flour and adding nutmeg, cloves, and melted butter. My dad loved the casserole so much that we ended up calling it "Cleve's casserole."

Dessert on Sundays was from Yvonne's Kitchen. My dad proudly hung a "Yvonne's Kitchen" plaque in our kitchen. He purchased the sign from a talented artisan in San Diego, who was selling her wares on the scenic shore overlooking Coronado. It's in our kitchen to this day. My mom would whip up a delectable homemade dessert, such as tiramisu, cheesecake, coffee cake, carrot cake, and zucchini bread. Occasionally, my dad would bake his signature cornmeal cake. Each golden slice revealed raisins studded throughout like tiny treasures, with bright red cherries crowning the top - a recipe he remains proud of.

Dinner party guests would often ask my mom where she bought the delicious rolls, cheesecake, or tiramisu. Before she could answer, my dad would proudly chime in, "Yvonne's Kitchen." Many assumed he was referring to a fancy, upscale bakery, only to be astonished when they discovered that these incredible treats were made right at home by my mom.

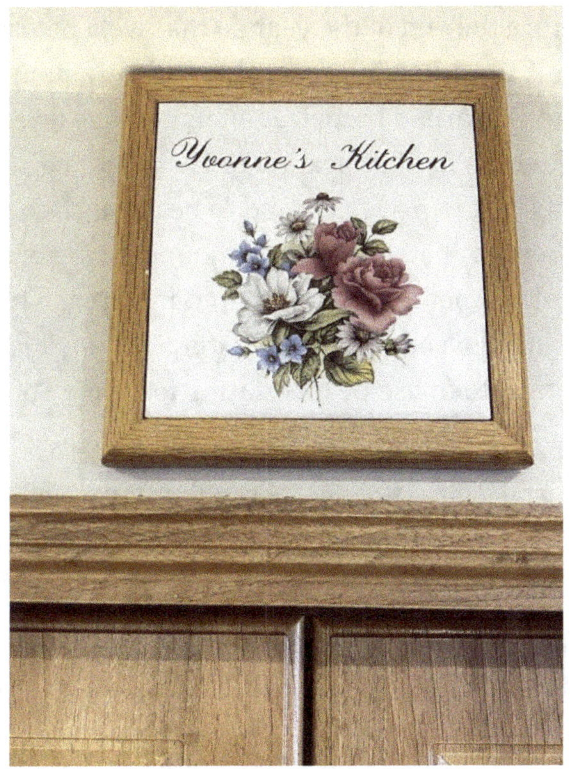

Plaque hanging in our kitchen for 20+ years

*** Samantha's Schooling ***

Being the first-born of twin girls, my educational journey started in the same manner as my sister's. I started junior kindergarten at Levy Creek Public School, but I don't have much memory of my one year at the school. However, what I do recall is Antoinette occasionally sneaking into my class during lunchtime. We are not conjoined twins, but we were practically joined at the hip growing up – and still are.

I then continued my education at Vista Heights Public School. I don't have much memory of senior kindergarten, but my mom ensured that my sister and I could read simple words and writing before the end of the year so that we'd be prepared to start Grade 1 the following year. Alongside my standard classes, my sister and I learned French at an immersive level which came in handy during a family vacation to Paris, France, many years later. During that trip, I was proud to be a translator for my parents. They, not being able to pronounce some of the French words, would sometimes ask that I put my French to use to order their meals. Today, like my sister, I put my high school French certificate to use by translating for some of my clients.

In second grade, I decided to join the school's cross-country team out of curiosity and discovered that I was naturally skilled at running. I placed in the top three in many of my cross-country meets from second grade to fifth grade.

Aside from physical activity, academics were always a priority, and an emphasis was placed on studying and homework at a young age. Throughout elementary school, my mom summer-schooled us, most intensely during the month of August. We would have daily English and Math lessons and concluded our summer break with a summer book report, which usually included a summary of our family vacation. This was done to give us a head start in the upcoming school year.

Those book reports inspired me, at just eight years old, to write my first novel. Though it remains unpublished, I hold onto the hope that it will find its way to readers someday. My journey with writing was a testament to the creative spark within me, even as a child.

Like my sister, I switched to Divine Mercy Catholic Elementary School for Grades 6 to 8. There, my French Immersion education transitioned to Core French. Being an active child, my love for athletics continued. At this stage of my life, I experienced playing in organized sports and competing against other schools for the first time. I played on the soccer team for one year and was on the basketball and volleyball teams during my three years at Divine Mercy. Our basketball and volleyball teams were very successful, as we added to our school's legacy by winning two championships.

My time at St. Aloysius Gonzaga Secondary School for Grades 9 to 12 was as eventful as my previous school years. I had the good fortune of being a part of the school band. I played the clarinet for 2 years and participated in school band performances. Like my sister and brother, I was also involved in student council through the Junior Leaders and Prefect programs. Athletics also continued in high school; I was a member of the volleyball and basketball teams, and in grade 12, I was awarded MVP and captain of the Senior Girl's Basketball team. All these activities led to a fruitful high school experience.

I took English in summer school every July at the end of Grades 9, 10, and 11, which allowed me to have spare periods in Grade 12. This was fortunate since I started University in May of 2019 while I was in my last semester of high school. This granted me the flexibility to use that spare period to work on my university materials. I eventually completed my law degree in November 2023.

Due to my active nature, I often experienced knee pain for most of my life, with the pain worsening as I became more and more active. Having previously been on several drugs to manage Severe Acute Aplastic Anemia, my mom took it upon herself to find an alternative to pharmaceuticals. She began researching natural, organic remedies to soothe my knee and muscle pain. After almost a year of trial and error, she created a unique formulation of pain-relieving organic essential oils to help with the pain and now sells this family recipe; she calls it komfiCare because it provides comfortable care. Today, it's available for others at www.komfiCare.com. My mom has jars of it within arm's reach on every bedside table and coffee table, and my dad even uses it daily for his mild degenerative arthritis. The use of komfiCare and physiotherapy sessions at Dr. Remy's clinic, The Chiropractic Office & Health Associates, helps me to continue to maintain a high level of physical activity.

I remain undeterred by the health challenges I have faced. Despite ongoing monitoring for Aplastic Anemia, I have learned to transform these obstacles into sources of hope, building a future filled with purpose and promise.

6

The Degrees

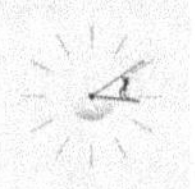

***** Cleveland's *****

After completing my A Levels in 1984, I applied to study computer science at the University of the West Indies (UWI), Mona campus in Jamaica. I was accepted; however, I did not have the financial means to attend. I deferred my application to the next year and found a job working at the Bank of Nova Scotia in Halfway Tree, Kingston. I continued to defer my acceptance for another two years.

I never attended UWI, Mona.

After migrating to Canada, I applied to the BSc in computer science program at York University, and in the autumn of 1995, I started classes in the part-time evening program. The first year was excellent. By the second year, I developed what is now called chronic fatigue syndrome – back then, my doctors didn't have a term to explain what was happening to me.

The frequent intense headaches, accompanied by dizziness and random joint pain, meant that I could not focus on writing my computer science C++ assignment codes. It also meant that I missed many hours at work because some days, I was just too dizzy to leave the house.

The family doctor that I had then gave me a good bit of advice that didn't include medication. "Cleveland, you need to scale

131

back your activities and put some joy in your life," she said. I was volunteering in church as a musician at the time while working fulltime and attending York part-time. So, I dropped all activities except work. I took some two weeks of vacation and spent in excess of five hours sleeping during the daytime for those two weeks. My bedtime routine was now changed to being in bed by 8:00 PM every night.

I did not complete the degree at York University.

By 2008, I regained my former energy and decided that once again. I would pursue the BSc in computer science that didn't want us to be joined together. This time around, I did not have the luxury of going to evening classes, and neither could I attend full-time because I was traveling heavily across North America as part of my job. If only I could find a distance learning program I wished. So, I went searching on the internet for any school in the world that offered a distance learning program.

I found distance learning programs in computer science that were offered by the University of London (UoL). I was very skeptical. My investigation revealed that it wasn't a university institution in the traditional sense, but rather, it was a federation of universities. The almost twenty federation members included the prestigious London School of Economics, Goldsmiths, King's College, London Business School, London School of Hygiene & Tropical Medicine, and Queen Mary University.

I also discovered that individuals such as Jamaica's Prime Minister Michael Manley and the globally influential Nelson Mandela earned degrees from the University of London schools.

This sealed my decision to study computer Science at this institution.

I submitted my application to study computer science; however, before starting, I changed my major to a BSc in Business Administration. This was heavily influenced by my own observations working for a large technology networking firm and the writings of authors such as Michio Kaku and Nicholas Carr's "The Big Switch." I became convinced that business acumen would be required to be linked with technical smarts for the future. Seeing that I had multiple technical certifications at this time and my career was progressing in the technical fields, I felt that I needed to bolster my knowledge of business. And if needs be, I would continue to grow my technical skills.

I started the BSc in Business Administration in 2009 via UoL's international distance learning program. I read books and completed coursework on flights, on weekends, and when at home, one hour of reading from 5:00 AM to 6:00 AM, Mondays to Fridays. I made the family room that sat atop the double car garage in our house my personal library. I had books and journal articles sprawled everywhere. Like the library, no one could walk safely in the room and not trip over books. I was fair to the family because I had an identical setup in the basement with a large-screen television and sound system, so they didn't miss any entertainment that they might have wanted.

In my late 40s, on March 19th, 2013, I attended my graduation ceremony at the Barbican Center in London, successfully completing a BSc from the University of London's Royal Holloway College.

At the graduation, I was told that a few students from the 3000+ graduating class were selected for a small reception. To my surprise, while the previously graduated students waited, in walked an entourage with The Princess Royal, Princess Anne. She graciously chatted and laughed with me about Jamaica, Canada, and the Caribbean in general. A collage of pictures from that event is in a later chapter of this book.

At the end of my BSc studies in 2012, I applied to read for a Master of Business Administration (MBA) at UoL's Royal Holloway College. I started the program in 2013. The MBA was part of the international distance learning program. However, it required traveling to the pristine sleepy town of Egham, in Surrey, UK, for two plenary sessions of lectures and other engagements with faculty and students. I attended the first plenary in July 2013 and the second in July 2014.

For my MBA dissertation, I chose to do primary research on the use of cloud computing by small businesses in Canada and how they match it with their business requirements. The dissertation was accepted and considered good enough that parts of it were published in a peer-reviewed journal. My co-author on that paper was my dissertation supervisor, Professor Harindranath.

In 2015, in my early 50s, I completed an MBA with Merit.

I owe much to Professor Harindranath's guidance during the writing of the fifteen-thousand-words dissertation and the two thousand-five-hundred-words published paper. The paper continues to be used by university students around the world today. A web search for "Cleveland Stanberry University of London" should find the paper.

Applying the principles of the MBA helped in tremendous ways to move my career into the business of consulting and was instrumental in giving me the competencies to provide analytical thought leadership that benefits clients' organizations.

*** **Yvonne's** ***

After attending Bloor Collegiate High School in Toronto, I enrolled, studied for, and, in 1993, successfully earned a Diploma in Business Administration and a Certificate in Human Resources Management from the Humber College of Applied Arts and Technology located in Toronto. After paying off my student loan I had hoped to continue studying to obtain a bachelor's degree. However, life's circumstances dictated otherwise.

By 2008, my visits to SickKids hospital were less frequent, and Samantha's platelet and other bloodlines were stable. Cleveland suggested that seeing that she is so stable, I should consider filling my days with a program of study from the University of London that would give me the bachelor's degree for which I hoped.

Great idea, I thought. I wrote an email requesting a printed university course prospectus. I combed through it as soon as I received it, and while there were many interesting degree courses, I wrestled with what was best for me.

By this time, I was volunteering at my children's school for the past five years. Based on the tasks that I was doing helping children in grades one and two to read, I felt that the knowledge gained would help me connect with what I was discovering, which was my passion for teaching young children.

The children that I helped were from varying home backgrounds, so I selected to apply to read for the BSc in Sociology. I figured that this would help me to better understand how to interact with these young learners.

The studying process was tiring. My study hours started when the children left for school and ended when they got home. After they arrived home, I pivoted into being a mother and a wife. Weekends were also no-study days. I remember how, on many days, I would walk around the street on which we lived, just crying my eyes out because I couldn't understand one or more statistical concepts. Chi-squared was one such concept. I spend hours, days and weeks trying to grasp the materials relating to statistical Chi-squared.

I knew I had to master Chi-squared before sitting UoL proctored exams that are held at the University of Toronto's Mississauga campus. Based on sample past questions provided by UoL, Chi-squared featured prominently as a main part of every former statistics exam.

My persistence paid off. Chi-squared eventually became one of the statistical concepts that I understood above and beyond all other concepts in the statistics course.

I passed my statistics exam.

Due to volunteering at the twin girl's school, if Samantha ever got sick and needed to be driven to SickKids within an hour, plus home management duties, I chose to take five years to complete the degree. However, unbeknownst to me when I made the decision, five years of study allowed Cleveland and I to synchronize our graduations on the same day.

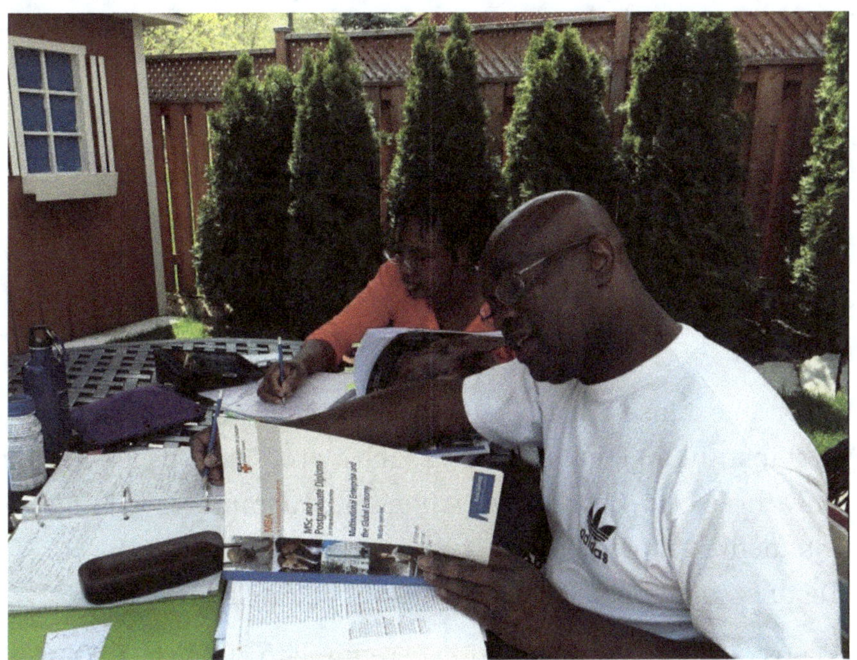

Yvonne & Cleveland studying on a usually warm spring day - on the patio in their backyard (May 2015)

Happily, on Tuesday, March 8th, 2016, at the Barbican Centre in London, I graduated with a BSc (honors) in Sociology, and he graduated with an MBA (Merit). A picture from that graduation ceremony with our children hovering over us is in a later chapter of this book. The link to UoL graduation ceremonies can be found by scanning this QR code below.

***** Clive-Anthony's *****

In 2019, I successfully earned my BSc in Mathematics and Economics from the London School of Economics. It seems my grade 6th teacher, Mr. McCaughey, could see shades of the future, as he thought that I would become an actuary, having performed so well in mathematics. Though the COVID-19 pandemic prevented a traditional graduation ceremony in 2020, I was already focused on my next goal: pursuing an MSc in Data Science.

After an extensive search, the University of London became the first institution I found offering such a program. Despite having only three courses available when the program was announced, I immediately applied and completed my MSc, earning a Distinction in Data Science and Artificial Intelligence in 2022.

I chose to defer my graduation ceremony to 2024 so that my sisters and I could graduate together - a decision likely influenced by my parents' practical consideration of not having the family of five traveling to graduations in London in consecutive years.

This educational foundation served me well in my career journey. I started as a data analyst with a large food manufacturer before being recruited by a media firm in London with offices overlooking the London Eye. I needed to relocate to take up this new role. However, delays caused by COVID-19 travel restrictions led to an unexpected turn when a major game developer in New York City offered me a position as a data scientist that didn't require immediate relocation. I accepted the data scientist role in New York City.

Today, I continue to work in New York City as a Data Quality Engineer at the National Football League (NFL), collaborating with coaches and health and safety professionals to ensure the well-being and safety of players. I continue to build upon the solid educational foundation that began with a simple, if slightly misleading, lesson about the importance of doing homework. Looking back, that "big lie" might have been unconventional parenting, but it sparked a drive for education that has shaped my entire life's trajectory.

***** Antoinette's *****

Since 9th grade, I had planned to pursue computer science, driven by my creativity and interest in engineering. However, in 2018, I discovered data science. The field's blend of computer programming and data-driven predictions captivated me, sparking a deeper interest. At that time, the University of London was the only institution I found offering a Bachelor of Science in Data Science. My cohort was the very first batch to study data science at the University of London International Programs.

I started university while still in High School, and from April to June of 2019, I had to juggle the requirements of both high school and university commitments. This was challenging, but I coped. To cope with the added stress, I joined the track team, running one and two hundred sprints as well as one hundred and four hundred meter hurdles.

I successfully completed my degree in computer science and data science, graduating with honors in 2024. Our mother's insistence on swimming lessons, which culminated in lifeguard and swimming instructor certifications, provided me with valuable skills for a lifeguard job that allowed me to pay my way through university without getting student loans and later being saddled with debt.

Today, I am fortunate to be working as a systems engineer, applying my passion for robotics to develop embedded code for Internet of Things hardware devices. My educational journey, shaped by both academic pursuits and extracurricular activities, has prepared me for a fulfilling career.

***** Samantha's *****

Looking back, I realize how important my upbringing was in shaping who I am. Our mom insisted that my siblings and I learn to swim, leading us all to become lifeguards. Saturdays were often spent at the community pool, where we learned skills that would serve us well. Lifeguarding not only taught me responsibility but also became a crucial source of income during my youth.

My financial independence grew further thanks to my dad, who shared his investment strategies with us. With lifeguarding income and strategic investments, I was able to pay for most of my university education with only minimal help from my parents.

I pursued a law degree inspired by a book my mom bought me while I was in grade 5. The book was titled Theodore Boone, Kid Lawyer, by John Grisham. The novel sparked my fascination with the legal profession. From that moment, I was determined that law would be my career path.

I completed an LLB with honors in 2023, choosing to study at the University of London because it gave me the lowest-cost route to a fast entry into the profession. Today, I am navigating the NCA process to become licensed and called to the Bar.

Currently, I work as a law clerk at a boutique law firm, focusing on wills and estates. I've also had the opportunity to work on cases in intellectual property, criminal law, and family law.

While I haven't yet decided which area of law I will specialize in, and because I have no student loans, I'm investing 90% of my earnings so that, hopefully, I will be able to fund my pathway to being called to the Bar.

7

The Lesson we learned

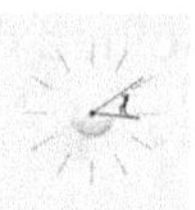

U p to this point for our family, the common theme that we might have been taught from life's journey is that no matter how challenging the circumstances that we experience might be, or how blissful the joys we experience and in which we revel, or indeed, how uncertain our planned futures might seem, it's never too late, sometimes.

Never too late it was to listen to that small, at times nagging voice, spurring us to act with our health or the health of someone about whom we care. Fortunately, Yvonne listened to the 'voice,' and because of that single obedience to act, above all else, it resulted in the survival of our daughter and sister Samantha.

Sometimes, it might never be too late at any age to learn something new. In his late 40s, Cleveland started and earned his first undergraduate degree. By his early 50s, he wound up walking the stage to collect the master's degree he earned. Not only did he earn the master's degree at what some might consider a late stage, but excerpts from his primary research paper ended up in a peer-reviewed published paper. Published by the Association for Information Systems, the paper can be found in the AIS Electronic Library by scanning the QR code below.

During the AIS conference Cleveland was offered to extend his research topic by completing a PhD. The offers came from the Universities of British Columbia on the west coast, and Queens University on the east coast (both in Canada). Cleveland pondered the offers and, in the end, to the utmost disgust of his son Clive-Anthony, he chose not to pursue a PhD. Clive-Anthony quipped, "you're breathing, so you can do it!". The timing didn't seem right for Cleveland and our family financial circumstances at the time. However, like a colleague of mine said, it might never be too late at any age to obtain a PhD, because his father completed his PhD at age 90. Is there hope for Cleveland?

Fortunate enough was Cleveland that at one of his graduation ceremonies, he was invited to a private reception with the chancellor of the University of London, Her Royal Highness, Princess Royal. Scan the QR code below to view pictures of the reception.

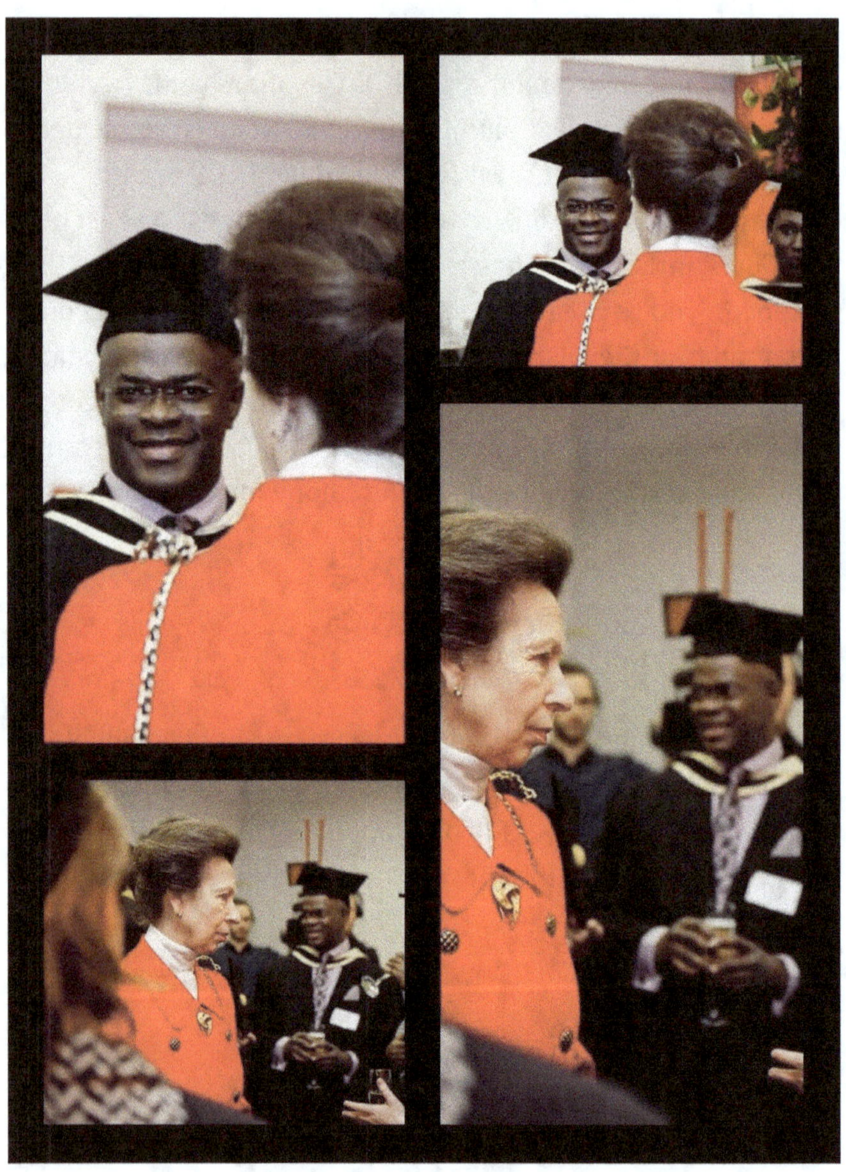

"Cleveland meeting HRH Princess Anne at his graduation in March 2013"

Sources:

https://www.flickr.com/photos/londoninternational/albums/7215763264433819/with/8658400476

https://www.london.ac.uk/current-students/graduation/past-ceremonies#:~:text=The%202016%20London%20Graduation%20Ceremony,at%20the%20Barbican%20Centre%2C%20London

It's never too late sometimes, for someone who yearned for an undergraduate degree after holding a college diploma to return to satisfy the desire. Yvonne earned an undergraduate degree in her late forties while balancing healthcare duties for her daughter, volunteering in her children's school, and being a stay-at-home mother and wife. It is this last degree that served as the springboard that allowed her to eventually launch her own tutoring business. It just so happened that Yvonne's late entry to enroll in her undergraduate degree led her and Cleveland to graduate at the same time, with a BSc in Sociology and him with an MBA. Their children joined them at their graduation, as depicted in the photo below.

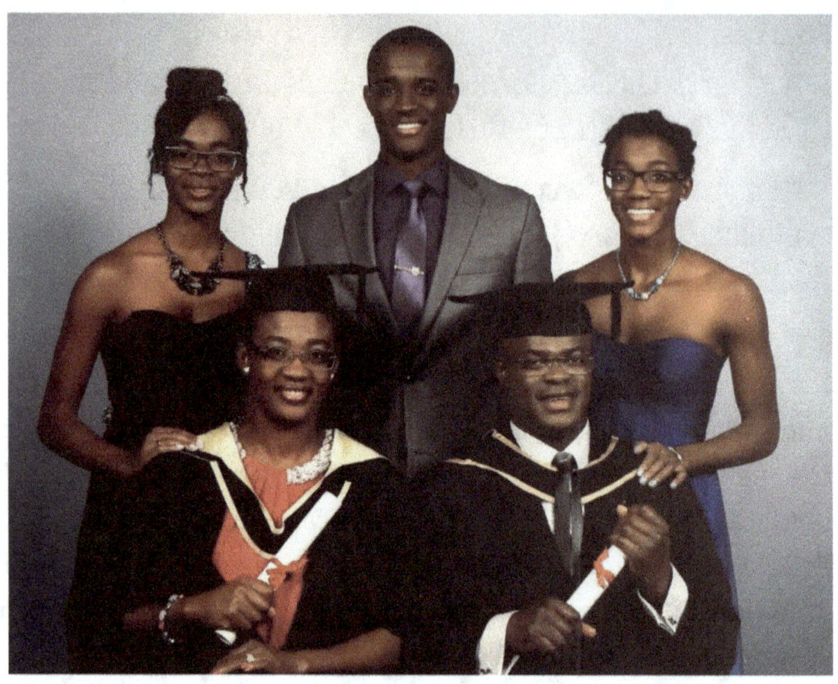

Parents' graduation in March 2016

*** 1 University, Family of 5, 7 Degrees ***

Even though Samantha suffered from her rare condition, it was never too late for her to join her siblings in engaging fully in sports activities as soon as she got the all-clear signal from her hematologist.

Now, the long-term outlook might be brighter for patients like Samantha, who suffered from Severe Aplastic Anemia and who were given immunosuppressive therapy (IST). In a 2023 Haematogica editorial published on the National Library of Medicine's website, the findings suggest that patients who survive after one year of IST can expect to live beyond five or ten years.

Samantha is incredibly blessed and fortunate to be part of that cohort of survivors. Remarkably, she has now reached twenty years of survival since completing her first year of immunosuppressive therapy!

More details can be read on the National Library of Medicine's website (https://pmc.ncbi.nlm.nih.gov/) by scanning the QR Code below.

As fate would have it, or as the circumstances that unfolded driven by the Covid pandemic, Samantha and her siblings all graduated together, where they shared the degrees of LLB, BSc Data Science and Computer Science, and Master of Artificial Intelligence and Data Science.

It just so happened that all five members of our family earned undergraduate and graduate degrees from the same university, the University of London. In total we hold seven degrees – two master's and five Bachelor's. Below is a photo of the children at their graduation in April 2024, accompanied by their parents.

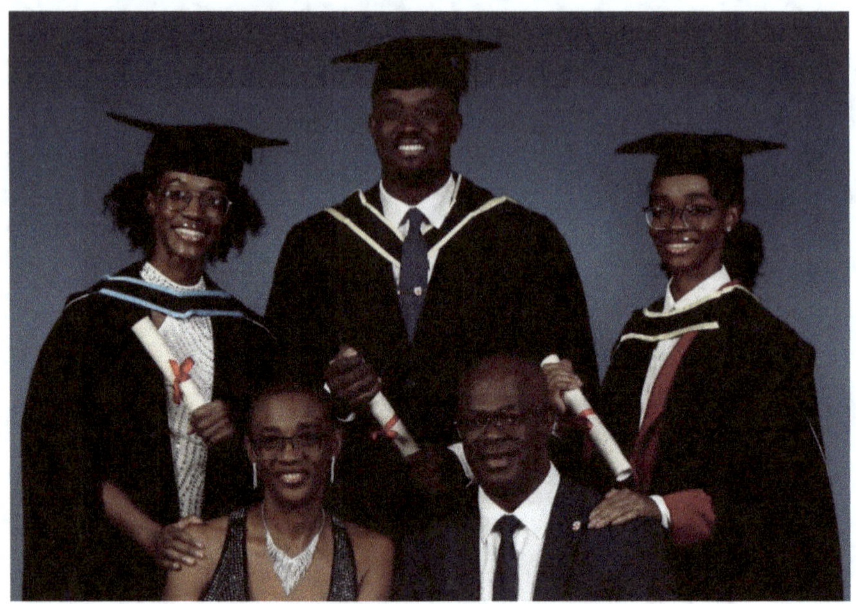

Children's graduation in April 2024

Our education journey was captured in two online articles by the University of London.

In the summer of 2016, Yvonne and Cleveland's academic journey with the university was documented based on an interview by Lisa Pierre, the head of alumni relations at the University's international program, in the magazine WC1E. The published magazine article can be read by scanning the QR code below.

The second publication of our family's academic journey by the university was eight years later, in the summer of 2024. This was in a University of London blog. It can be read by scanning the QR code below.

It's never too late to dream of what could be done to propel us from where we are in life's journey to a path that is beneficial to us; Beneficial to our health and well-being. A path that serves in meaningful ways, a path that brings us closer to where we can see a glimpse of the hopes and dreams of the bright future that we all aspire to achieve. Indeed, it is a path that delivers us to those dreams that ultimately turn some of our visions into the reality that we desire.

While enjoying sumptuous meals at the dining table, since the early 2000s, we have discussed and contemplated over and over the writing of this book, so now it is our hope that in the autumn of 2024, we can state in concert that "it's never too late to write these words and share them with the world."

About The Authors

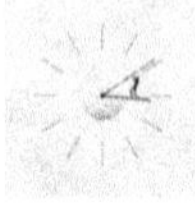

Yvonne is a dedicated mother, wife, and entrepreneur with a deep passion for early education. Her commitment to helping young children thrive led her to teach each of her children to recognize letters and numbers by age two, allowing them to read simple words before entering junior kindergarten. Leveraging her Diploma in Business Administration, Certificate in Human Resources, a University of London BSc with honors in Sociology, and a certificate from the University of Reading, UK, in "Supporting Successful Learning in Primary School," Yvonne transformed this passion into founding an online tutoring company, "To Learn is Empowering." Her company specializes in enhancing the abilities of young minds, particularly those facing learning challenges made more difficult by Fetal Alcohol Spectrum Disorder (FASD) and Attention Deficit Hyperactivity Disorder (ADHD). Through her work, Yvonne continues to make a meaningful impact in the lives of children who need support in reaching their academic potential. She's an avid reader of 19th and 20th-century romance British novels.

Samantha obtained an LLB with honors from the University of London and is currently working as a law clerk at a boutique law firm. The firm specializes in various fields, including Wills and Estates, Real Estate, Family, and Corporate Law. Samantha has a particular interest in Wills and Estates, where she dedicates her full efforts to support the department. Aspiring to become a lawyer in the future, Samantha enjoys arts and crafts during her downtime.

Antoinette holds a BSc with honors in Computer Science and Data Science from the University of London. In her role, she helps drive innovative AI applications that enhance customer interaction and experience. Antoinette is committed to continuous learning, regularly enrolling in online certificate courses to expand her knowledge and skills, both for her career and personal growth. Outside of work, she channels her creativity into painting and game development.

Clive-Anthony is a Data Quality Engineer in the Player Health & Safety division at the National Football League (NFL). He earned a Distinction in an MSc in Data Science and Artificial Intelligence from the University of London and a BSc in Mathematics and Economics from the London School of Economics. He specializes in enhancing data accuracy and fostering collaboration among athletic trainers and management across all NFL clubs. Clive-Anthony engineered and maintained the NFL Data Quality & Compliance Portal, assisting trainers & biomedical groups to keep high data quality standards. He is a regular speaker at technology and education conferences such as the Carnegie Mellon Sports Analytics Conference and the Canadian Edtech Summit, where he speaks about the intersectionality of quantitative findings informed by Data Science and AI on sports & education technologies. He enjoys spending his weekends playing basketball and pickleball.

Cleveland is passionate about aligning technology with business imperatives. He worked as a program manager, leading transformational projects in data science and cloud technologies to help organizations enhance and sustain their operational efficiencies and enhance their competitive advantages. He holds a BSc with honors and an MBA with merit from the University of London. He earned a Certificate in data science issued jointly by the University of Toronto School of Continuing Education and the University of Waterloo. From MIT Sloan School of Management, he holds a certificate in Artificial Intelligence (AI). He makes annual donations to support Sick Kids Hospital. A multi-instrumentalist, Cleveland enjoys playing smooth jazz on his keyboard or bass or streaming his favorite artists in his free time.

Heartfelt Thank You from
The Stanberry Archives ©

Dear readers, we understand that you have many choices when it comes to your reading pleasure.

This makes us immensely appreciative that you took the time to read our book. We are deeply grateful that you chose to embark on this journey of reflection that helped to discover that it's never too late, sometimes.

It is our hope that you too have been inspired to reflect on your past circumstances, and that somehow, those have now become the catalyst to drive you to personal discoveries.

We sincerely hope that the insights shared in this book have enriched your understanding of how unknown illnesses can be devastating, sometimes.

 We also trust that you have been encouraged to act on your own intuition when they arise.

Your feedback means so much to us. In the event something resonated with you, we kindly invite you to leave a review on Amazon. With appreciation, we thank you in advance.

9 798302 653918